Male Infertility

Editor

JAMES M. HOTALING

UROLOGIC CLINICS OF NORTH AMERICA

www.urologic.theclinics.com

Consulting Editor
SAMIR S. TANEJA

May 2020 • Volume 47 • Number 2

ELSEVIER

1600 John F. Kennedy Boulevard • Suite 1800 • Philadelphia, Pennsylvania, 19103-2899

http://www.theclinics.com

UROLOGIC CLINICS OF NORTH AMERICA Volume 47, Number 2
May 2020 ISSN 0094-0143, ISBN-13: 978-0-323-71207-1

Editor: Kerry Holland
Developmental Editor: Julia McKenzie

Urologic Clinics of North America (ISSN 0094-0143) is published quarterly by Elsevier Inc., 360 Park Avenue South, New York, NY 10010-1710. Months of issue are February, May, August, and November. Business and Editorial Offices: 1600 John F. Kennedy Blvd., Suite 1800, Philadelphia, PA 19103-2899. Periodicals postage paid at New York, NY and additional mailing offices. Subscription prices are $391.00 per year (US individuals), $795.00 per year (US institutions), $100.00 per year (US students and residents), $450.00 per year (Canadian individuals), $993.00 per year (Canadian institutions), $100.00 per year (Canadian students/residents), $520.00 per year (foreign individuals), $993.00 per year (foreign institutions), and $240.00 per year (foreign students/residents). Foreign air speed delivery is included in all *Clinics* subscription prices. All prices are subject to change without notice. **POSTMASTER:** Send address changes to *Urologic Clinics of North America*, Elsevier Health Sciences Division, Subscription Customer Service, 3251 Riverport Lane, Maryland Heights, MO 63043. **Customer Service: 1-800-654-2452 (US). From outside the United States, call 1-314-447-8871. Fax: 1-314-447-8029. E-mail: JournalsCustomerService-usa@elsevier.com (for print support)** and **JournalsOnlineSupport-usa@elsevier.com (for online support).**

Reprints. For copies of 100 or more, of articles in this publication, please contact the Commercial Reprints Department, Elsevier Inc., 360 Park Avenue South, New York, New York 10010-1710. Tel.: 212-633-3874; Fax: 212-633-3820; E-mail: reprints@elsevier.com.

Urologic Clinics of North America is covered in MEDLINE/PubMed (*Index Medicus*), *Excerpta Medica, Current Contents/Clinical Medicine, Science Citation Index,* and *ISI/BIOMED*.

Contributors

CONSULTING EDITOR

SAMIR S. TANEJA, MD
The James M. Neissa and Janet Riha Neissa Professor of Urologic Oncology, Professor of Urology, Radiology, and Biomedical Engineering, GU Program Leader, Perlmutter Cancer Center, Director, Division of Urologic Oncology, Department of Urology, NYU Langone Health, New York, New York, USA

EDITOR

JAMES M. HOTALING, MD, MS, FECSM
Associate Professor of Surgery (Urology), Adjunct Associate Professor of OBGYN, University of Utah School of Medicine, University of Utah Center for Reconstructive Urology and Men's Health, Salt Lake City, Utah, USA

AUTHORS

JASON P. AKERMAN, MD, FRCSC
Clinical Fellow, Department of Urology, The University of North Carolina at Chapel Hill, Chapel Hill, North Carolina, USA

PHILIP J. CHENG, MD
Reproductive Medicine Associates of New Jersey, Basking Ridge, New Jersey, USA; Division of Urology, University of Utah School of Medicine, Salt Lake City, Utah, USA

JEREMY T. CHOY, MD
Clinical Fellow, Endocrinology, Department of Medicine, Stanford University School of Medicine, Stanford, California, USA

ROBERT MATTHEW COWARD, MD, FACS
Associate Professor, Department of Urology, The University of North Carolina at Chapel Hill, Chapel Hill, North Carolina, USA; Director of Male Reproductive Medicine and Surgery, UNC Fertility, Raleigh, North Carolina, USA

SHERIN DAVID, PhD
Department of Obstetrics, Gynecology and Reproductive Sciences, Molecular Genetics and Developmental Biology Graduate Program, Magee-Womens Research Institute, University of Pittsburgh School of Medicine, Pittsburgh, Pennsylvania, USA

JAMES M. DUPREE, MD, MPH
Departments of Urology, Obstetrics and Gynecology, University of Michigan, Ann Arbor, Michigan, USA

MICHAEL L. EISENBERG, MD
Director, Male Reproductive Medicine and Surgery, Associate Professor, Departments of Urology and Obstetrics and Gynecology, Stanford University School of Medicine, Stanford, California, USA

JASON M. FRANASIAK, MD
HCLD/ALD, IVI-RMA New Jersey, Sidney Kimmel Medical College, Thomas Jefferson University, Basking Ridge, New Jersey, USA

JOSEPH SCOTT GABRIELSEN, MD, PhD
Department of Urology, University of Rochester Medical Center, Rochester, New York, USA

NICOLÁS GARRIDO, PhD, MSc
Director of IVI Foundation, Director of Research Administration at IVI RMA Global, Fundación Instituto Valenciano de Infertilidad (FIVI), Instituto Universitario IVI (IUIVI), Valencia, Spain

KELLI X. GROSS, MD
Division of Urology, Department of Surgery, University of Utah, Salt Lake City, Utah, USA

MATHEW M. GROVER
Department of Physiology and Developmental Biology, Brigham Young University, Provo, Utah, USA

BRENT M. HANSON, MD
IVI-RMA New Jersey, Sidney Kimmel Medical College, Thomas Jefferson University, Basking Ridge, New Jersey, USA

SOLOMON HAYON, MD
Resident, Department of Urology, The University of North Carolina at Chapel Hill, Chapel Hill, North Carolina, USA

IRENE HERVÁS, MSc
PhD Student, Fundación Instituto Valenciano de Infertilidad (FIVI), Instituto Universitario IVI (IUIVI), Valencia, Spain

JAMES M. HOTALING, MD, MS, FECSM
Associate Professor of Surgery (Urology), Adjunct Associate Professor of OBGYN, University of Utah School of Medicine, University of Utah Center for Reconstructive Urology and Men's Health, Salt Lake City, Utah, USA

KEITH JARVI, MD, FRCSC
Professor, Division of Urology, Department of Surgery, Institute of Medical Science, University of Toronto, Lunenfeld-Tannenbaum Research Institute, Mount Sinai Hospital, Toronto, Ontario, Canada

TIMOTHY G. JENKINS, PhD
Department of Physiology and Developmental Biology, Brigham Young University, Provo, Utah, USA

AKASH A. KAPADIA, MD
Department of Urology, University of Washington, Seattle, Washington, USA

DANIEL J. KASER, MD
IVI-RMA New Jersey, Sidney Kimmel Medical College, Thomas Jefferson University, Basking Ridge, New Jersey, USA

LARRY I. LIPSHULTZ, MD
Scott Department of Urology, Baylor College of Medicine, Houston, Texas, USA

ERIC M. LO, BS
Baylor College of Medicine, Houston, Texas, USA

SARAH C. McGRIFF, BS
Baylor College of Medicine, Houston, Texas, USA

AKANKSHA MEHTA, MD, MS
Assistant Professor, Department of Urology, Emory University School of Medicine, Atlanta, Georgia, USA

MUJALLI MHAILAN MURSHIDI, MD, FRCS (England)
Professor of Urology, The University of Jordan, Amman, Jordan; Visiting Scholar, Department of Urology, Stanford University School of Medicine, Stanford, California, USA

KYLE E. ORWIG, PhD
Department of Obstetrics, Gynecology and Reproductive Sciences, Molecular Genetics and Developmental Biology Graduate Program, Magee-Womens Research Institute, University of Pittsburgh School of Medicine, Pittsburgh, Pennsylvania, USA

ALEXANDER W. PASTUSZAK, MD, PhD
Division of Urology, Department of Surgery, University of Utah School of Medicine, Salt Lake City, Utah, USA

UJVAL ISHU PATHAK, MPH
Scott Department of Urology, Baylor College of Medicine, Houston, Texas, USA

MARY OAKLEY STRASSER, BA
Department of Urology, University of Michigan, Ann Arbor, Michigan, USA

CIGDEM TANRIKUT, MD, FACS
Shady Grove Fertility, Rockville, Maryland, USA; Department of Urology, Georgetown University School of Medicine, Washington, DC, USA

THOMAS J. WALSH, MD, MS
Associate Professor, Department of Urology, University of Washington, Seattle, Washington, USA

Contents

Preface: Male Infertility: Is It the Key to the Future of Reproductive Health? **xiii**

James M. Hotaling

Cutting-Edge Evaluation of Male Infertility **129**

Ujval Ishu Pathak, Joseph Scott Gabrielsen, and Larry I. Lipshultz

A male factor is a contributor in 50% of cases of infertility. Although assisted reproductive techniques can often bypass the need to improve semen parameters, the evaluation of the infertile man remains critical. Current methods for evaluating the infertile man are discussed, beginning with the basic workup that all suspected infertile men should undergo, followed by subsequent evaluation steps. Although the fundamental components of the evaluation have remained consistent, several new tools are available to assist in identifying the underlying etiology. As our understanding of male fertility expands, the technologies available to diagnose and ultimately treat it continue to evolve.

Optimal Endocrine Evaluation and Treatment of Male Infertility **139**

Sarah C. McGriff, Eric M. Lo, James M. Hotaling, and Alexander W. Pastuszak

This article aims to define the optimal endocrine workup of male factor infertility, including evaluation and treatment of men who have previously been on exogenous testosterone or anabolic steroids. Future directions include the expansion of genetic testing for infertility to include endocrine gene products.

Sperm Extraction in Obstructive Azoospermia: What's Next? **147**

Jason P. Akerman, Solomon Hayon, and Robert Matthew Coward

For men with obstructive azoospermia, several surgical sperm retrieval techniques can facilitate conception with assisted reproductive technology. The evolution of both percutaneous and open approaches to sperm retrieval has been affected by technological innovations, including the surgical microscope, in vitro fertilization, and intracytoplasmic sperm injection. Further modifications to these procedures are designed to minimize patient morbidity and increase the quality and quantity of sperm samples. Innovative technologies promise to further ameliorate outcomes by selecting the highest quality sperm. Although various approaches to surgical sperm retrieval are now well established, several advancements in sperm selection and optimization are being developed.

Testicular Mapping: A Roadmap to Sperm Retrieval in Nonobstructive Azoospermia? **157**

Akash A. Kapadia and Thomas J. Walsh

Guiding a couple with nonobstructive azoospermia requires an integrated approach to care by the urologist and the reproductive endocrinologist. After informing the couple of the implications of the diagnosis, care must be taken to outline the options of parenthood. Most experts agree that sperm retrieval in men can be challenging. This article describes various options of sperm retrieval, historic and contemporary, and highlights the advantages and disadvantages of each. The authors find that using a testicular map can invariably help guide sperm retrieval and overall fertility care. The right approach is one that involves a shared decision with the couple.

High Sperm DNA Damage: Does Testicular Sperm Make Sense? **165**

Keith Jarvi

Sperm DNA damage reduces pregnancy rates in couples undergoing in vitro fertilization (IVF). Because it has been shown that testicular sperm have lower DNA damage than ejaculated sperm, it is an attractive idea to consider using testicular sperm for IVF for men with high sperm DNA damage. In fact, there are multiple centers throughout the world now offering sperm retrieval for IVF to manage this condition. However, there is insufficient evidence to conclude that testicular sperm improves pregnancy/live birth rates. Further studies are required before offering sperm retrieval as a standard of care to manage high sperm DNA damage.

Round Spermatid Injection **175**

Kelli X. Gross, Brent M. Hanson, and James M. Hotaling

From a fertility perspective, men with azoospermia represent a challenging patient population. When no mature spermatozoa are obtained during a testicular sperm extraction, patients are often left with limited options, such as adoption or the use of donor sperm. However, it has been reported that round spermatids can be successfully injected into human oocytes and used as an alternative to mature spermatozoa. This technique is known as round spermatid injection (ROSI). Despite the limitations of ROSI and diminished clinical success rates, the use of round spermatids for fertilization may have potential as a treatment modality for men with azoospermia.

The Role of the Urologist in a Reproductive Endocrinology and Infertility Practice **185**

Philip J. Cheng and Cigdem Tanrikut

With male factor infertility accounting for up to 50% of infertility cases, demand for male fertility services has increased. Integrating a reproductive urologist within a fertility center allows for treatment of both partners simultaneously with easier, more convenient access to a comprehensive male evaluation and any indicated interventions. A joint practice allows urologists to collaborate more closely with reproductive endocrinologists, which can, in turn, improve clinical care and research endeavors. This full-service, streamlined approach translates to optimized care for the infertile couple and allows for emphasis of male partner health.

Care Delivery for Male Infertility: The Present and Future **193**

Mary Oakley Strasser and James M. Dupree

Although infertility is now recognized as a disease by multiple organizations including the World Health Organization and the American Medical Association, private insurance companies rarely include coverage for infertility treatments. In this review, the authors assess the current state of care delivery for male infertility care in the United States. They discuss the scope of male infertility as well as the unique burdens it places on patients and review emerging market forces that could affect the future of care delivery for male infertility.

Qualitative Research in Male Infertility 205

Akanksha Mehta

Qualitative research methods represent a valuable tool for investigating the entirety of the experience of male infertility evaluation, diagnosis, and treatment. Qualitative research is rigorous and thorough and well adapted for studying the complex field of infertility and reproductive health. Knowledge gained from qualitative research methods can undoubtedly inform clinical practice and improve support for individuals and couples affected by male factor infertility.

Male Infertility and Somatic Health 211

Mujalli Mhailan Murshidi, Jeremy T. Choy, and Michael L. Eisenberg

Somatic health is associated with male infertility; potential links between infertility and health may arise from genetic, developmental, and lifestyle factors. Studies have explored possible connections between male infertility and oncologic, cardiovascular, metabolic, chronic, and autoimmune diseases. Male infertility also may be a predictor of hospitalization and mortality. Additional research is required to elucidate the mechanisms by which male infertility affects overall health.

Transgenerational Epigenetics: A Window into Paternal Health Influences on Offspring 219

Mathew M. Grover and Timothy G. Jenkins

Transgenerational epigenetic inheritance provides a mechanism by which environmental exposures and lifestyle decisions can affect the offspring directly through the gamete. It is this pattern of inheritance that has shed light on the fact that preconception lifestyle decisions that a father makes are significant because they can significantly impact the offspring. Understanding the epigenetic alterations in gametes and the potential implications of these changes is key to the health of future generations.

Spermatogonial Stem Cell Culture in Oncofertility 227

Sherin David and Kyle E. Orwig

Infertility caused by chemotherapy or radiation treatments negatively impacts patient-survivor quality of life. The only fertility preservation option available to prepubertal boys who are not making sperm is cryopreservation of testicular tissues that contain spermatogonial stem cells (SSCs) with potential to produce sperm and/or restore fertility. SSC transplantation to regenerate spermatogenesis in infertile adult survivors of childhood cancers is a mature technology. However, the number of SSCs obtained in a biopsy of a prepubertal testis may be small. Therefore, methods to expand SSC numbers in culture before transplantation are needed. Here we review progress with human SSC culture.

Personalized Medicine in Infertile Men 245

Nicolás Garrido and Irene Hervás

Personalized medicine gathers the most relevant data involved in human health. Currently, the diagnosis of male infertility is limited to spermiogram, which does not provide information on the male fertile potential. New diagnostic methods are required. The application of omics techniques in the study of male reproductive health renders a huge amount of data providing numerous novel infertility

UROLOGIC CLINICS OF NORTH AMERICA

FORTHCOMING ISSUES

August 2020
Cancer Immunotherapy in Urology
Sujit S. Nair and Ashutosh Tewari, *Editors*

November 2020
Advanced and Metastatic Renal Cell Carcinoma
William C. Huang, Ezequiel Becher, *Editors*

February 2021
Robotic Urology: The Next Frontier
Jim C. Hu and Jonathan Shoag, *Editors*

RECENT ISSUES

February 2020
Salvage therapies for Non-Muscle Invasive Bladder Cancer
Badrinath R. Konety, *Editor*

November 2019
Gender Affirming Surgery
Lee C. Zhao, Rachel Bluebond-Langner, *Editors*

August 2019
Modern Management of Testicular Cancer
Sia Daneshmand, *Editor*

Preface

Male Infertility: Is It the Key to the Future of Reproductive Health?

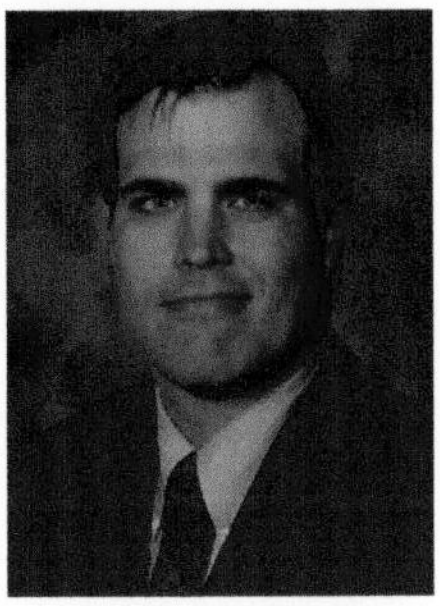

James M. Hotaling, MD, MS, FECSM
Editor

Male infertility is a common and devastating disease. Despite the advances in the field, we still struggle to identify, diagnose, and treat this condition. Furthermore, the field of reproductive urology trails at least 20 years behind that of female infertility. With 1% of children in the United States now born through in vitro fertilization and up to 2% to 3% in Europe, some recent high-profile papers highlighting declining sperm counts around the world, and other data linking male infertility to poor individual and familial somatic health, it is vital that we focus our efforts on understanding this disease.

Fortunately, the future for our field looks bright. The articles written here serve to demonstrate the tremendous recent advances to address these issues as well as to provide a glimpse of what the future might hold. One analogy that serves to highlight the cusp of the revolution that our field is currently standing on is that of oncology. Currently, aspects of male infertility are roughly where cancer was at the advent of chemotherapy and targeted radiation. At the advent of these treatments, we did not understand the fundamental biology of specific tumors, did not have databases to track outcomes, poorly understood what patients' goals of treatment were, did not have broad insurance coverage of these treatments, and, hence, could not offer targeted therapies that optimized outcomes and helped patients achieve their goals. Now we understand the biology of specific tumors and have tied this to robust data in clinical outcomes. This has allowed a revolution in diagnostic tools. Furthermore, insight into the fundamental biology of various subtypes of cancer has facilitated a number of new medical therapies, checkpoint inhibitors being 1 example. Similar advances in male infertility have the potential to impact not only infertile men but also their families as well as global health through the reduction in transmission of deleterious genetic and epigenetic variants to offspring and grand-offspring.

While male infertility is certainly much further along than cancer at the advent of therapeutic agents such as cisplatin, the lack of clear understanding of the biology, epidemiology, pathogenesis, and health services research implications of the disease has hampered transformative research in the field. These articles highlight some of the most promising areas of male infertility and, it is hoped, convince the reader that the future of our field has never been brighter.

James M. Hotaling, MD, MS, FECSM
University of Utah School of Medicine
1012 North East Capitol Boulevard
Salt Lake City, UT 84103, USA

E-mail address:
Jim.Hotaling@hsc.utah.edu

Urol Clin N Am 47 (2020) xiii
https://doi.org/10.1016/j.ucl.2020.01.002

Cutting-Edge Evaluation of Male Infertility

Ujval Ishu Pathak, MPH[a], Joseph Scott Gabrielsen, MD, PhD[b], Larry I. Lipshultz, MD[a,*]

KEYWORDS

• Male infertility • Semen analysis • Physical examination • Genetic testing • Epigenetics

KEY POINTS

- A male factor contributes to 50% of cases of infertility, yet only 7.5% of men are referred for urologic evaluation.
- The male infertility evaluation is critical to identify the cause of infertility but may also reveal other information relevant to the health of the patient and his offspring.
- The history, physical, and semen analysis remain the mainstay of the male infertility evaluation. Additional hormonal and genetic testing may be indicated.

INTRODUCTION

Infertility affects up to 15% of the world's population, with approximately half involving a male factor.[1,2] The inability to conceive can have impacts on patients' self-esteem, mental health, financial status, and even their marriages. Beyond the direct effects of infertility however, there are indirect associations of infertility with a man's health that highlight the importance of a fertility evaluation for every man. Factors contributing to infertility can range from the easily correctible (eg, changing timing of intercourse) to the currently irreversible. For example, up to 10% of the infertile couples with male factor infertility may have reversible causes such as varicoceles or obstruction.[3] Consequently, any investigation into a couple's infertility should thoroughly evaluate the male partner.

Traditionally, infertility has been defined as the inability of a man and woman to conceive after 12 months of unprotected intercourse.[4] An infertility evaluation is recommended after 6 months, however, if the woman is older than 35 years.[5] Couples are increasingly delaying attempts at conceiving until after career development, resulting in progressively later attempts at pregnancy, and apprehension surrounding their potential fertility often prompts requests for earlier workups. Although no laboratory test can guarantee that a couple is fertile, prompt evaluation can identify problems that can guide their planning.

Spermatogenesis and fertilization are complex processes involving a combination of genetic, hormonal, environmental, and other factors, and failure of any of these can result in infertility. Because of this, the goals of a thorough infertility workup are manifold. The primary goals are to identify the etiology of the infertility, and determine whether it is reversible and whether there are contributing factors that may impact the patient's overall health. Timely addressing a reversible etiology such as gonadotoxic exposure or an underlying medical condition can often result in rapid improvement of fertility.[6,7] If an irreversible etiology is uncovered, the physician should determine whether the condition is amenable to assisted reproductive technologies (ARTs) (eg, intrauterine insemination [IUI] or in vitro fertilization [IVF] with intracytoplasmic sperm injection [ICSI]). If not,

[a] Scott Department of Urology, Baylor College of Medicine, 6624 Fannin Street, Suite 1700, Houston, TX 77030, USA; [b] Department of Urology, University of Rochester Medical Center, 601 Elmwood Avenue, Box 656, Rochester, NY 14642, USA
* Corresponding author. Scott Department of Urology, Baylor College of Medicine, 6624 Fannin Street, Suite 1700, Houston, TX 77030.
E-mail address: larryl@bcm.edu

Urol Clin N Am 47 (2020) 129–138
https://doi.org/10.1016/j.ucl.2019.12.001

then the patient may need to consider adoption or use of donor sperm. It is also important to identify genetic etiologies that may be passed on to the patient's offspring, warranting referral to genetic counseling.

The increasing prevalence and availability of IVF and other ARTs have greatly enhanced the ability of couples to have children. As only relatively few sperm are needed with ICSI, however, the male infertility evaluation is often skipped if there are sufficient sperm in the ejaculate for ART. Thus, fewer than 40% of subfertile men undergo evaluation.[8] This is particularly concerning, however, as male infertility may be associated with other underlying disease states. For example, infertile men have a higher risk of cancer, immune problems, cardiovascular disease, and overall mortality.[9–11] Without an infertility workup, these potentially life-threatening conditions for which infertility is a symptom may go unnoticed and the opportunity for early diagnosis missed. Thus, even if couples are planning ART due to a known female factor, the male partner also should undergo a comprehensive evaluation if semen quality is impaired.

Despite a thorough investigation, a male etiology will escape a specific diagnosis in 15% to 30% of cases.[12] Recent advances in the diagnostic workup for male factor infertility have increased our understanding and ability to diagnose contributing factors. The goal of this article is to provide an up-to-date guide to the diagnostic workup of the infertile man and highlight advances in the field that may greatly expand our ability to diagnose and treat these men in the future.

BASIC EVALUATION

A thorough medical history, physical examination, and at least 2 semen analyses are the cornerstone of any evaluation of the infertile man.[4] These provide information that can guide treatment and further evaluation.

History and Physical Examination

The workup for infertility begins with the history and physical. Emphasis should be placed on interviewing the couple. A comprehensive approach to history taking involves inquiring about reproductive, sexual, medical, surgical, infectious disease, childhood conditions, and gonadal toxin exposure history. Stress also should be discussed, as it may contribute to impaired fertility and sexual dysfunction.[13,14] Discussion should focus on present attempts at conceiving, timing of intercourse, and use of lubricants, as well as the menstrual history and previous evaluation of the female partner. Whether either partner has previously caused/been pregnant also should be noted. Essential components of the history are listed in **Table 1**.

Family history is an increasingly important part of the patient's history given the genetic basis of infertility. The X chromosome has many genes critical to spermatogenesis. As men normally have a single copy of the X chromosome, any mutation in these genes can affect male fertility, as there is no second chromosome to compensate,[15] whereas female individuals with a mutated copy may still be fertile. Thus, men should be asked about family history of infertility, particularly in brothers and maternal uncles, as this may indicate

Table 1
History components of the male infertility evaluation

Category	Components
Reproductive history	Past attempts at conceiving Previous treatments for infertility Birth control Sexual technique and lubricants Timing of intercourse Previous pregnancies Menstrual history and female evaluation
Sexual history	Erectile dysfunction Hypogonadism Ejaculatory dysfunction Sexually transmitted disease
Medical history	Fevers or systemic illness Diabetes Spinal cord injury
Gonadotoxins	Drugs (exogenous anabolic steroids, tobacco/nicotine exposure, alcohol, narcotics, marijuana, immunosuppressants, chemotherapy) Radiation exposure Pesticides Thermal exposure Testosterone or steroids
Surgical history	Hernia repair Scrotal trauma Testicular torsion Varicocele repair Orchiopexy Transurethral resection of prostate
Family history	Infertility Genetic disorders Consanguinity

an X-linked genetic transmission. Given the elevated risk of cancers among infertile men,[10,16] history of cancers in first-degree and second-degree relatives should also be identified. Other significant illnesses in family members (eg, cystic fibrosis) also should be noted.

Physical examination should begin with gross assessment of general appearance, body habitus, and secondary sexual characteristics. Findings such as gynecomastia or gynecoid hair distribution may be indicative of underlying endocrine or genetic abnormalities. Likewise, obesity can be associated with lower testosterone and an abnormal testosterone-to-estradiol ratio.[17] Penile anatomy, such as penile curvature or plaques and location of the urethral meatus also should be inspected, as these abnormalities can impair sexual intercourse or result in an inability for ejaculate to reach the cervix, respectively. A careful examination of the scrotal contents and inguinal region should be done. Close attention should be paid to abnormal testis volume or consistency, the presence of varicoceles, and, specifically, the presence of both vasa deferentia and epididymides.

A physical examination is critically important, as findings may identify or rule out potential etiologies of infertility. Most testicular volume is composed of the seminiferous tubules, thus, abnormal testes size and consistency suggest impaired spermatogenesis, and may indicate androgen deficiency. Absence of one or both vasa should raise concern for cystic fibrosis (further discussed in "Radiological Examination" and "Cystic Fibrosis Gene Mutations"), and induration of the epididymides in the presence of normal-sized testicles is suggestive of obstruction.[18] Pertinent findings on physical examination can be found in **Table 2**. A digital rectal examination (DRE) also should be considered to examine the prostate and to check for midline cysts or enlarged seminal vesicles. Any abnormal findings on DRE should prompt a transrectal ultrasound (TRUS).

Table 2
Physical examination components of the male infertility evaluation

Category	Findings
General	Body habitus Gynecomastia Gynecoid features
Penis	Meatus location (hypospadias or epispadias) Curvature (chordee/Peyronie disease) Ulceration (venereal disease)
Testes	Size (endocrine disorder) Consistency Contours and masses (malignancy)
Epididymides	Cysts Spermatocele
Vasa deferentia	Atresia or agenesis (cystic fibrosis) Granuloma
Spermatic cords	Asymmetry Varicocele
Rectal examination	Midline cysts Dilated seminal vesicles Enlarged prostate

Semen Analysis

The semen analysis it the key laboratory test in the evaluation of the infertile man. Collection of the semen should be done after the patient has been abstinent for 2 to 5 days, as sperm concentration, volume, and motility may be affected by shorter and longer abstinence periods. Semen samples are usually collected by masturbation in the clinic; however, if masturbation is not possible for religious or other reasons, the patient may use specialized seminal collection condoms. Samples collected at home should be kept at room or body temperature and brought to the clinic within 1 hour. At least 2 analyses are recommended, as there is often variation between different analyses of the same individual.[19] When there are highly divergent analyses, a third sample is required to determine the baseline for that individual. **Table 3** contains the reference values based on data from the World Health Organization.

It should be noted that the reference values are statistically determined and do not reflect "normal" values. The values are based on the 95th percentile of parameters of men with proven fertility.[19] Thus, 5% of the fertile population would be expected to fall below the lower reference limit. Semen parameters of infertile men overlap considerably with those of fertile men. In addition, "normal" semen analyses are found in more than 40% of couples undergoing fertility evaluation,[20] suggesting although sperm are necessary for fertilization, the presence of sperm does not guarantee fertility. Likewise, low semen parameters generally do not guarantee infertility.

Semen volume abnormalities, such as aspermia (total absence of semen) or seminal hypovolemia (<1.0 mL), may point to specific anatomic factors as a cause of infertility. These findings may be the result of functional issues, such as retrograde ejaculation, or anatomic variations, such as

Table 3
World Health Organization semen analysis reference ranges (5th edition)

Parameter	Lower Reference Limit (95% Confidence Interval)
Semen volume, mL	1.5 (1.4–1.7)
Total sperm number, 10^6/ejaculate	39 (33–46)
Sperm concentration, 10^6/mL	15 (12–16)
Total motility, %	40 (38–42)
Progressive motility, %	32 (31–34)
Sperm morphology, normal forms, %	4 (3.0–4.0)

Data from World Health Organization. WHO laboratory manual for the examination and processing of human semen. 5th ed. Geneva: World Health Organization; 2010.

ejaculatory ductal obstruction or hypoplasia of the prostate or seminal vesicles due to congenital bilateral absence of the vasa deferentia (CBAVD) or androgen deficiency, respectively. If the vasa are palpable bilaterally, a postejaculatory urinalysis should be obtained to determine whether retrograde ejaculation is present. TRUS can be used to visualize the seminal vesicles and prostate to determine whether ejaculatory duct obstruction (dilated seminal vesicles), hypoplastic seminal vesicles (seen in CBAVD), or other structural abnormalities may be causing obstruction (eg, prostatic cysts).

Sperm concentrations less than 15 million/mL define oligozoospermia.[21] Absence of sperm from the ejaculate is azoospermia; however, this can be diagnosed only if the semen sample has been centrifuged and the pellet found to lack sperm.[19] Sperm concentrations less than 10 million/mL should prompt endocrine testing, whereas concentrations less than 5 million/mL should prompt genetic testing.[4] An increased sensitivity in genetic testing is found when one limits testing to less than 1 million, but this may increase missed positive findings.

Asthenozoospermia, or impaired sperm motility, is another potential hindrance to fertility, as sperm progression is requisite for natural fertilization. The 3 categories of motility are progressive (comprising all sperm moving in a linear or circular pattern), nonprogressive, and immotile; the latter 2 consisting of all sperm that do not progress. In some conditions (eg, Kartagener syndrome), the sperm may be uniformly immotile. Vitality testing can be used to differentiate alive but immotile sperm from necrozoospermia (ie, all dead sperm).[19] The total motile sperm count (concentration * volume * percent motility) is often used clinically; this calculated result is most useful to determine what degree of assisted reproduction may be needed.

Sperm morphology refers to the shape of the spermatozoa, with the lower reference limit in fertile men being 4% normal forms.[19] Thus, even in fertile men, the vast majority of sperm have abnormal morphology. The definition of normal morphology has become progressively stricter in each of the 5 editions of the World Health Organization guidelines. Meta-analyses have demonstrated, however, that abnormal sperm morphology using the current guidelines does not predict IUI, IVF, or ICSI success,[22,23] and thus the true significance of this number has been called into question. Indeed, Kovac and colleagues[24] demonstrated that among 24 men with severe teratozoospermia (ie, 0% normal morphology), 25% were subsequently able to conceive naturally.

Zero percent normal forms should not be confused, however, with 100% of sperm showing the same abnormal morphology. These diseases, such as globozoospermia, are usually associated with genetic abnormalities. Most of these patients have extremely low success rates of natural and assisted conception, although some may be amenable to modifications of the ICSI procedures (eg, ICSI success rates are improved with oocyte activation in globozoospermia due to *DPY19L2* mutations[25]). Others, such as macrocephalic sperm, have high rates of aneuploidy.[26] As genetic testing for these conditions is not routine, men with these types of abnormal morphology should be referred for genetic counseling.

Testosterone and Follicle-Stimulating Hormone

Approximately 3% of cases of male infertility are attributable to endocrine problems.[27] It is recommended that testosterone and follicle-stimulating hormone levels be measured as part of an endocrine evaluation in men with sperm counts of less than 10 million/mL or if there are features on physical examination suggestive of endocrine dysfunction.[4] The endocrine evaluation of infertile men is covered in more detail in Sarah C. McGriff and colleagues' article, "Optimal Endocrine Evaluation and Treatment of Male Infertility," elsewhere in this issue. Based on the physical examination, semen analyses, and endocrine testing, further testing may be indicated.

EXTENDED EVALUATION

Radiological Examination

Scrotal, transrectal, and renal ultrasonography are generally not part of the initial evaluation of male infertility, but may be useful adjuncts to better delineate anatomy and identify potential etiologies.

Although varicocele is typically a clinical diagnosis, scrotal ultrasound can be used to objectively measure varicocele vein diameters and document reversal of blood flow with Valsalva.[28] Ultrasonography can be particularly useful in individuals whose body habitus makes physical examination difficult or in individuals with a history of varicocele repair; however, ultrasound is not necessary in most situations. Scrotal ultrasound should be performed if there is a testicular mass or if hydroceles, scarring, or other factors making direct palpation of the testicles difficult on physical examination. A recent publication, however, calls into question the suitability of surgery for subclinical varicoceles, showing the same increase in total motile count when comparing results of clinical and subclinical varicocele repair results.[29]

Transrectal ultrasound (TRUS) is used to evaluate abnormal DRE findings or to assess in the diagnosis of ejaculatory duct obstruction in patients with low semen volume.[30] TRUS enables visualization of enlarged seminal vesicles or cysts at the ejaculatory ducts, which may be the source of anejaculation, hematospermia, or painful ejaculation. Seminal vesicle aspiration is often used concurrently. In cases of CBAVD, TRUS also may be used to assess hypoplasia or agenesis of the seminal vesicles.[3] The vasa deferentia can be identified on TRUS, thus this can also be used if their presence is unclear on physical examination.

Renal and urinary tract ultrasonography are used less frequently, but they are indicated in cases of CBAVD and unilateral absence of the vas deferens to rule out unilateral renal agenesis, which is found in 10% and 25% of these patients, respectively.[31]

MRI of the pituitary fossa is indicated in men found to have elevated prolactin levels or unexplained hypogonadotropic hypogonadism during endocrine evaluation to rule out pituitary adenoma (see Sarah C. McGriff and colleagues' article, "Optimal Endocrine Evaluation and Treatment of Male Infertility," elsewhere in this issue). Less commonly, pelvic MRI can be used to identify the internal accessory organs; however, TRUS is usually sufficient and less expensive.

Laboratory Assessment

Depending on the sperm concentration or suspected etiology, genetic testing or sperm integrity testing (eg, seminal oxidant levels, DNA fragmentation, fluorescence in situ hybridization (FISH)) may be indicated.

Karyotype testing

A karyotype is recommended in men who have a sperm concentration less than 5 million/mL and should be considered if there is suspicion for numerical chromosome abnormalities (eg, Klinefelter syndrome) or large structural abnormalities (eg, translocations, deletions).[4] Chromosomal abnormalities are identified more frequently as sperm concentrations decrease: karyotypic abnormalities are found in fewer than 1% of men with normal sperm parameters, ~5% of men with severe oligospermia, and 10% to 15% of men with azoospermia.[32,33] Kleinfelter syndrome (XXY) is the most common chromosomal abnormality associated with male infertility.

Balanced translocations can result in phenotypically normal men; however, failure of meiotic pairing of the chromosomes can result in decreased sperm concentrations and sperm with imbalanced translocations. Thus, the male partner in couples with recurrent pregnancy loss should also have a karyotype performed.[4] As chromosomal abnormalities can potentially be passed on to offspring, men with chromosomal abnormalities should be referred for genetic counseling before consideration of ART.

Y chromosome microdeletion testing

Y chromosome microdeletion (YCMD) testing is indicated in men who have sperm concentrations less than 5 million/mL. Seven percent of men with impaired spermatogenesis have microdeletions of regions of their Y chromosome compared with 2% of normozoospermic men.[34] YCMDs are classified by regions called azoospermia factor regions (AZFa, AZFb, and AZFc). Depending on the region of the microdeletion, the outcome can range from moderate impairment of spermatogenesis to complete azoospermia. These regions are too small to be detected with karyotype testing and require polymerase chain reaction amplification of sites within each region. Complete AZFa and/or AZFb deletions are incompatible with spermatogenesis, and men with these deletions should not undergo attempts at testicular sperm extraction.[35] Spermatogenesis can occur in men with AZFc deletions, however, and azoospermic men with these deletions have approximately 50% likelihood of having sperm on microsurgical testicular sperm extraction.[36] YCMDs affect the Y chromosome and will be passed on to 100% of their male offspring, so men with YCMDs should meet with a genetic counselor before pursuing ART.

Cystic fibrosis gene mutations

Cystic fibrosis is due to mutations in the *CFTR* gene on chromosome 7. CBAVD is present in all men with clinical symptoms of cystic fibrosis; however, approximately 80% of men with CBAVD have mutations in the *CFTR* gene even in the absence of respiratory manifestations of the disease.[37] Thus, patients with CBAVD should undergo *CFTR* gene testing regardless of whether they have pulmonary manifestations of cystic fibrosis. Complete *CFTR* gene sequencing should be considered in all ethnic minorities with CBAVD given higher rates of less common variants. Congenital unilateral absence of the vas deferens (CUAVD) is variably associated with mutations in the *CFTR* gene.[37] Individuals with CUAVD should undergo renal ultrasound due to a high percentage having renal agenesis on the ipsilateral side, yet not necessarily associated with *CFTR* mutations.[31] Patients with these mutations should receive genetic counseling, and their partner should be tested given the relatively high prevalence of *CFTR* mutation carriers in the general population.

Seminal oxidants

Reactive oxygen species (ROS) are naturally produced by oxidative reactions. ROS play a critical role in the sperm acrosomal reaction; however, polyunsaturated fatty acids in the sperm membrane are particularly susceptible to oxidation by ROS, resulting in impaired sperm motility and DNA damage.[38–40] Elevated ROS levels are found in men with a variety of impaired semen parameters and may be a contributing factor in 25% to 40% of men.[41–43] ROS testing can be challenging, however, as not all laboratories have the necessary equipment. In addition, specimens must be tested shortly after ejaculation, as antioxidants in the seminal plasma may quench the ROS.

DNA fragmentation

Sperm lack mechanisms for DNA repair and, therefore, accumulate DNA damage as they pass through the reproductive tract. Although there is robust DNA repair on fertilization, excess DNA damage can prevent embryo development. Direct assays of DNA fragmentation measure the number of breaks in DNA, whereas indirect assays measure the sensitivity of DNA to acid-induced denaturation.[4] Higher levels of DNA fragmentation are seen as sperm counts decrease and are associated with IVF failure.[44,45] Thus, DNA fragmentation testing should be considered in individuals planning ART and those who have had unexplained recurrent pregnancy loss. Some studies have shown superior DNA quality in testicular sperm compared with ejaculated sperm.[46]

Fluorescence in situ hybridization

Sperm are normally haploid, containing a single copy of the 22 autosomes and an X or Y chromosome. Errors in meiotic segregation, however, can result in aneuploid sperm. As many as 6% of infertile men have elevated levels of aneuploid sperm.[47] Depending on the chromosome, sperm aneuploidy can result in viable embryos (eg, Klinefelter syndrome, Down syndrome, Turner syndrome); however, gain or loss of most chromosomes are incompatible with life. Thus, men with a high number of aneuploid sperm are at risk for recurrent pregnancy loss or fetal abnormalities. Sperm FISH can be used to identify the percentage of aneuploid sperm; however, there are currently few centers offering this testing.

Advanced Testing/Future Directions

Our understanding of male fertility continues to evolve at a rapid rate, and now includes important roles for genetics, epigenetics, metabolomics, and extracellular vesicle function. Each new discovery, however, highlights how much we have yet to understand and discover. Although not currently part of the recommended testing, diagnostic and therapeutic advances in these fields may bring them to the forefront of the male infertility evaluation in the upcoming years.

Additional Genetic Testing

Testing for *CFTR* mutations in men with CBAVD is currently the only specific gene recommended by guidelines. This traditionally has been due to the cost of sequencing and the relative infrequency of specific mutations in the general infertile population. Nonetheless, men with specific phenotypes could benefit from additional genetic testing and referral to a genetic counselor should be considered. These potentially significant genes include *ADGRG2* testing in men with *CFTR* mutation-negative CBAVD[48]; *DPY19L2*, *PICK1*, or *SPATA16* testing in men with globozoospermia[49–51]; or *AURKC* in men with macrocephalic sperm with multiple flagella.[52] Easily identifiable characteristics such as these may increase the yield of genetic testing in specific populations.

Alternatively, the rapidly decreasing cost and increasing throughput of next generation sequencing technologies has allowed for sequencing of entire panels of genes, and even whole exome and whole genome sequencing, well below the traditional cost of sequencing a single gene. For example, a targeted panel sequencing 87 genes previously associated with male and female infertility cost only $599 and had nearly 100% accuracy for detecting mutations and sex chromosome aneuploidies and 94% accuracy for YCMD.[53] These targeted sequencing technologies are also amenable to benchtop sequencers, facilitating integration into the andrology laboratory of the future. Thus, targeted or more extensive sequencing may ultimately become part of standard infertility testing.

Epigenetics

DNA modifications such as methylation (the most common type of epigenetic modification) can silence gene expression without altering the fundamental genetic sequence. Indeed, epigenetic modifications allow cell type–specific gene expression despite all cells sharing the same genetic code. Thus, abnormal methylation could silence genes in a spermatogonial stem cell or other germ cell, resulting in infertility. Abnormal epigenetic modifications, or epimutations, are harder to detect than genetic mutations, as they may be cell type specific. To test for epigenetics, DNA from the target tissue (eg, testes) is needed, limiting the usefulness of current testing. Sperm DNA methylation has been studied, and global methylation has been shown to increase with age and is altered in male infertility.[54,55] As there is high heterogeneity of sperm DNA methylation within a single sample, however, the clinical utility of sperm methylation testing remains unclear.[56] Nonetheless, as epimutations are potentially reversible, further research may allow for identification of epimutation-driven male infertility and targeted treatment to reverse it.

Metabolomics, Proteomics, Lipidomics, and Other "-omics"

Genetic mutations and epimutations can affect gene expression and protein function, ultimately altering the production of metabolites and other factors necessary for spermatogenesis and fertility. Metabolomics, on the other hand, focuses on the concentrations of the metabolites within a sample to identify factors that may be associated with disease, and secondarily assesses the pathways that may be contributing to the abnormal concentration. Similarly, proteomics can identify protein concentrations, lipidomics, lipid concentrations, and so forth. This can be particularly advantageous, as there may be many pathways converging and diverging from a specific metabolite or other factor, and the ultimate concentration of one or more substances may contribute more to infertility than a specific pathway. Thus, these studies often identify molecular signatures of disease that can subsequently be developed into biomarkers for diagnostic purposes.

As metabolomics looks at metabolite concentrations, it is naturally inclined to look at the production and consumption of metabolites, the most common of which are often involved in energy production. Thus, metabolomic analysis in male infertility has often focused on men with asthenozoospermia, as altered energy production can contribute to decreased motility.[57] One challenge with this approach, however, is that although molecular signatures can be identified for asthenozoospermia, there is limited clinical utility for that information. For example, a molecular signature was identified in the seminal plasma of men with asthenozoospermia compared with controls, and when converted to an algorithm, the signature accurately predicted the motility of 5 of 6 subjects.[58] Standard semen analysis, however, is sufficient to classify asthenozoospermia from normozoospermia.

Other similar types of studies have highlighted the challenges in trying to use metabolomic and other molecular concentrations as a basis to treat disease. Altered concentrations of a substrate may be the cause of infertility; however, it may also just be a by-product of some other reaction. Thus, correcting the abnormal signature may not improve fertility. For example, lipidomics have identified that seminal plasma and sperm docosahexaenoic acid (DHA) levels decrease with worsening semen parameters.[59] A double-blind, placebo-controlled trial of DHA supplementation in men with infertility failed to improve motility or count in asthenozoospermic men.[60] Thus, whether the low DHA is impairing motility, or whether it is simply a by-product of another process remains unclear. Nonetheless, as molecular signatures for infertility become better defined, these may be amenable to targeted interventions in the future.

Extracellular Vesicles

Exosomes and other extracellular vesicles are secreted by cells and can transmit RNAs, proteins, metabolites, and other substances. Extracellular vesicles produced by the epididymis (also known as, epididymosomes) have been shown to play an important role in sperm maturation by delivering protein cargos to the sperm as they transit the epididymis.[61] Exosomes in the seminal plasma have been shown to affect sperm motility.[62] Exosomes and other extracellular vesicles are found throughout the male and female reproductive tract. We are just beginning to understand the critical and complex role they play in male fertility.[63]

SUMMARY

The proper evaluation of the male is a critical component of the evaluation of the infertile couple. Despite advances in ART that permit paternity with a limited number of sperm, the purpose of the examination of the infertile man goes beyond identifying the cause of infertility and may identify factors that could affect the health of the patient and/or his offspring. Although the fundamental components of the evaluation have remained constant, advances in our understanding of the pathophysiology, combined with advances in technology, have enhanced our ability to diagnose and treat male infertility.

ACKNOWLEDGMENTS

J.S. Gabrielsen was supported in part by National Institutes of Health grant K12 DK083014 (Multidsciplinary K12 Urologic Research [KURe] Career Development Program awarded to Dolores J. Lamb) and the Winfield Scott Charitable Trust.

REFERENCES

1. Agarwal A, Mulgund A, Hamada A, et al. A unique view on male infertility around the globe. Reprod Biol Endocrinol 2015;13:37.
2. Thonneau P, Marchand S, Tallec A, et al. Incidence and main causes of infertility in a resident population (1,850,000) of three French regions (1988-1989). Hum Reprod 1991;6(6):811–6.
3. Esteves SC, Miyaoka R, Agarwal A. An update on the clinical assessment of the infertile male. [corrected]. Clinics (Sao Paulo) 2011;66(4):691–700.
4. Practice Committee of the American Society for Reproductive Medicine. Diagnostic evaluation of the infertile male: a committee opinion. Fertil Steril 2015;103(3):e18–25.
5. Practice Committee of the American Society for Reproductive Medicine. Definitions of infertility and recurrent pregnancy loss: a committee opinion. Fertil Steril 2013;99(1):63.
6. Smith RP, Coward RM, Lipshultz LI. The office visit. Urol Clin North Am 2014;41(1):19–37.
7. Hsieh TC, Pastuszak AW, Hwang K, et al. Concomitant intramuscular human chorionic gonadotropin preserves spermatogenesis in men undergoing testosterone replacement therapy. J Urol 2013; 189(2):647–50.
8. Chandra A, Copen CE, Stephen EH. Infertility service use in the United States: data from the National Survey of Family Growth, 1982-2010. Natl Health Stat Report 2014;(73):1–21.
9. Skakkebaek NE, Rajpert-De Meyts E, Buck Louis GM, et al. Male reproductive disorders and fertility trends: influences of environment and genetic susceptibility. Physiol Rev 2016;96(1):55–97.
10. Hanson BM, Eisenberg ML, Hotaling JM. Male infertility: a biomarker of individual and familial cancer risk. Fertil Steril 2018;109(1):6–19.
11. Glazer CH, Bonde JP, Eisenberg ML, et al. Male infertility and risk of nonmalignant chronic diseases: a systematic review of the epidemiological evidence. Semin Reprod Med 2017;35(3):282–90.
12. Practice Committee of the American Society for Reproductive Medicine. Effectiveness and treatment for unexplained infertility. Fertil Steril 2006;86(5 Suppl 1):S111–4.
13. Nordkap L, Jensen TK, Hansen AM, et al. Psychological stress and testicular function: a cross-sectional study of 1,215 Danish men. Fertil Steril 2016;105(1):174–87.e1-2.
14. Song SH, Kim DS, Yoon TK, et al. Sexual function and stress level of male partners of infertile couples during the fertile period. BJU Int 2016;117(1):173–6.
15. Ropke A, Tuttelmann F. Mechanisms in Endocrinology: aberrations of the X chromosome as cause of male infertility. Eur J Endocrinol 2017;177(5): R249–59.
16. Eisenberg ML, Betts P, Herder D, et al. Increased risk of cancer among azoospermic men. Fertil Steril 2013;100(3):681–5.
17. Bieniek JM, Kashanian JA, Deibert CM, et al. Influence of increasing body mass index on semen and reproductive hormonal parameters in a multi-institutional cohort of subfertile men. Fertil Steril 2016;106(5):1070–5.
18. Schoor RA, Elhanbly S, Niederberger CS, et al. The role of testicular biopsy in the modern management of male infertility. J Urol 2002;167(1):197–200.
19. World Health Organization. WHO laboratory manual for the examination and processing of human semen. 5th edition. Geneva (Switzerland): World Health Organization; 2010.
20. van der Steeg JW, Steures P, Eijkemans MJ, et al. Role of semen analysis in subfertile couples. Fertil Steril 2011;95(3):1013–9.
21. Cooper TG, Noonan E, von Eckardstein S, et al. World Health Organization reference values for human semen characteristics. Hum Reprod Update 2010;16(3):231–45.
22. Kohn TP, Kohn JR, Ramasamy R. Effect of sperm morphology on pregnancy success via intrauterine insemination: a systematic review and meta-analysis. J Urol 2018;199(3):812–22.
23. Hotaling JM, Patel DP, Vendryes C, et al. Predictors of sperm recovery after cryopreservation in testicular cancer. Asian J Androl 2016;18(1):35–8.
24. Kovac JR, Smith RP, Cajipe M, et al. Men with a complete absence of normal sperm morphology exhibit high rates of success without assisted reproduction. Asian J Androl 2017;19(1):39–42.

25. Eskandari N, Tavalaee M, Zohrabi D, et al. Association between total globozoospermia and sperm chromatin defects. Andrologia 2018;50(2).
26. Carmignac V, Dupont JM, Fierro RC, et al. Diagnostic genetic screening for assisted reproductive technologies patients with macrozoospermia. Andrology 2017;5(2):370–80.
27. Sigman M, Jarow JP. Endocrine evaluation of infertile men. Urology 1997;50(5):659–64.
28. Chiou RK, Anderson JC, Wobig RK, et al. Color Doppler ultrasound criteria to diagnose varicoceles: correlation of a new scoring system with physical examination. Urology 1997;50(6):953–6.
29. Thirumavalavan N, Scovell JM, Balasubramanian A, et al. The impact of microsurgical repair of subclinical and clinical varicoceles on total motile sperm count: is there a difference? Urology 2018;120:109–13.
30. Shefi S, Turek PJ. Definition and current evaluation of subfertile men. Int Braz J Urol 2006;32(4):385–97.
31. Schlegel PN, Shin D, Goldstein M. Urogenital anomalies in men with congenital absence of the vas deferens. J Urol 1996;155(5):1644–8.
32. Ravel C, Berthaut I, Bresson JL, et al. Genetics Commission of the French Federation of CECOS. Prevalence of chromosomal abnormalities in phenotypically normal and fertile adult males: large-scale survey of over 10,000 sperm donor karyotypes. Hum Reprod 2006;21(6):1484–9.
33. Van Assche E, Bonduelle M, Tournaye H, et al. Cytogenetics of infertile men. Hum Reprod 1996; 11(Suppl 4):1–24 [discussion: 25–6].
34. Pryor JL, Kent-First M, Muallem A, et al. Microdeletions in the Y chromosome of infertile men. N Engl J Med 1997;336(8):534–9.
35. Hopps CV, Mielnik A, Goldstein M, et al. Detection of sperm in men with Y chromosome microdeletions of the AZFa, AZFb and AZFc regions. Hum Reprod 2003;18(8):1660–5.
36. Oates RD, Amos JA. The genetic basis of congenital bilateral absence of the vas deferens and cystic fibrosis. J Androl 1994;15(1):1–8.
37. Casals T, Bassas L, Ruiz-Romero J, et al. Extensive analysis of 40 infertile patients with congenital absence of the vas deferens: in 50% of cases only one CFTR allele could be detected. Hum Genet 1995;95(2):205–11.
38. Aitken RJ, Paterson M, Fisher H, et al. Redox regulation of tyrosine phosphorylation in human spermatozoa and its role in the control of human sperm function. J Cell Sci 1995;108(Pt 5):2017–25.
39. Aitken RJ, Gordon E, Harkiss D, et al. Relative impact of oxidative stress on the functional competence and genomic integrity of human spermatozoa. Biol Reprod 1998;59(5):1037–46.
40. Griveau JF, Le Lannou D. Reactive oxygen species and human spermatozoa: physiology and pathology. Int J Androl 1997;20(2):61–9.
41. Padron OF, Brackett NL, Sharma RK, et al. Seminal reactive oxygen species and sperm motility and morphology in men with spinal cord injury. Fertil Steril 1997;67(6):1115–20.
42. de Lamirande E, Gagnon C. Impact of reactive oxygen species on spermatozoa: a balancing act between beneficial and detrimental effects. Hum Reprod 1995;10(Suppl 1):15–21.
43. Aitken RJ, Buckingham D, West K, et al. Differential contribution of leucocytes and spermatozoa to the generation of reactive oxygen species in the ejaculates of oligozoospermic patients and fertile donors. J Reprod Fertil 1992;94(2):451–62.
44. Borges E Jr, Zanetti BF, Setti AS, et al. Sperm DNA fragmentation is correlated with poor embryo development, lower implantation rate, and higher miscarriage rate in reproductive cycles of non-male factor infertility. Fertil Steril 2019;112(3):483–90.
45. Yılmaz S, Zergeroğlu AD, Yılmaz E, et al. Effects of sperm DNA fragmentation on semen parameters and ICSI outcome determined by an improved SCD test, Halosperm. Int J Fertil Steril 2010;4(2): 73–8.
46. Greco E, Scarselli F, Iacobelli M, et al. Efficient treatment of infertility due to sperm DNA damage by ICSI with testicular spermatozoa. Hum Reprod 2005; 20(1):226–30.
47. Egozcue S, Blanco J, Vendrell JM, et al. Human male infertility: chromosome anomalies, meiotic disorders, abnormal spermatozoa and recurrent abortion. Hum Reprod Update 2000;6(1): 93–105.
48. Patat O, Pagin A, Siegfried A, et al. Truncating mutations in the adhesion G protein-coupled receptor G2 gene ADGRG2 cause an X-linked congenital bilateral absence of vas deferens. Am J Hum Genet 2016;99(2):437–42.
49. Dam AH, Koscinski I, Kremer JA, et al. Homozygous mutation in SPATA16 is associated with male infertility in human globozoospermia. Am J Hum Genet 2007;81(4):813–20.
50. Liu G, Shi QW, Lu GX. A newly discovered mutation in PICK1 in a human with globozoospermia. Asian J Androl 2010;12(4):556–60.
51. Elinati E, Kuentz P, Redin C, et al. Globozoospermia is mainly due to DPY19L2 deletion via non-allelic homologous recombination involving two recombination hotspots. Hum Mol Genet 2012;21(16): 3695–702.
52. Dieterich K, Soto Rifo R, Faure AK, et al. Homozygous mutation of AURKC yields large-headed polyploid spermatozoa and causes male infertility. Nat Genet 2007;39(5):661–5.
53. Patel B, Parets S, Akana M, et al. Comprehensive genetic testing for female and male infertility using next-generation sequencing. J Assist Reprod Genet 2018;35(8):1489–96.

54. Jenkins TG, Aston KI, Cairns B, et al. Paternal germ line aging: DNA methylation age prediction from human sperm. BMC Genomics 2018;19(1):763.
55. Denomme MM, McCallie BR, Parks JC, et al. Alterations in the sperm histone-retained epigenome are associated with unexplained male factor infertility and poor blastocyst development in donor oocyte IVF cycles. Hum Reprod 2017;32(12):2443–55.
56. Laurentino S, Beygo J, Nordhoff V, et al. Epigenetic germline mosaicism in infertile men. Hum Mol Genet 2015;24(5):1295–304.
57. Zhao K, Zhang J, Xu Z, et al. Metabolomic profiling of human spermatozoa in idiopathic asthenozoospermia patients using gas chromatography-mass spectrometry. Biomed Res Int 2018;2018:8327506.
58. Gilany K, Moazeni-Pourasil RS, Jafarzadeh N, et al. Metabolomics fingerprinting of the human seminal plasma of asthenozoospermic patients. Mol Reprod Dev 2014;81(1):84–6.
59. Zerbinati C, Caponecchia L, Rago R, et al. Fatty acids profiling reveals potential candidate markers of semen quality. Andrology 2016;4(6):1094–101.
60. Conquer JA, Martin JB, Tummon I, et al. Effect of DHA supplementation on DHA status and sperm motility in asthenozoospermic males. Lipids 2000;35(2):149–54.
61. Nixon B, De Iuliis GN, Hart HM, et al. Proteomic profiling of mouse epididymosomes reveals their contributions to post-testicular sperm maturation. Mol Cell Proteomics 2019;18(Suppl 1):S91–108.
62. Murdica V, Giacomini E, Alteri A, et al. Seminal plasma of men with severe asthenozoospermia contain exosomes that affect spermatozoa motility and capacitation. Fertil Steril 2019;111(5):897–908.e2.
63. Gabrielsen JS, Lipshultz LI. Rapid progression in our understanding of extracellular vesicles and male infertility. Fertil Steril 2019;111(5):881–2.

Optimal Endocrine Evaluation and Treatment of Male Infertility

Sarah C. McGriff, BS[a], Eric M. Lo, BS[a], James M. Hotaling, MD, MS, FECSM[b], Alexander W. Pastuszak, MD, PhD[b,*]

KEYWORDS

• Male • Infertility • Endocrine • Hypogonadism • Anabolic steroid • Testosterone • Genetic testing

KEY POINTS

- Endocrinopathies that affect male fertility are rare, but important to consider as causes of male factor infertility and should be screened for in the initial history and physical examination.
- Classification of hormonal abnormalities by their effect on the hypothalamic-pituitary-testicular axis and the potential for reversibility guides evaluation and treatment.
- The endpoint for treatment is stimulation of spermatogenesis, usually through hormonal pharmacology to raise the intratesticular concentration of testosterone.
- Precision medicine and genetic testing will likely become standard for infertility evaluation in the future, as more candidate genes for infertility are identified.

Endocrinopathies are uncommon etiologies of male factor infertility. The incidence of primary hormonal disorders as the cause of male infertility ranges from less than 1% to 3%.[1–3] Nonetheless, endocrine disorders are important to consider in the infertility evaluation, as up to 70% of men with infertility have concurrent endocrine dysfunction.[4] Metabolic syndrome, which is characterized by insulin resistance with hyperinsulinemia and obesity, has deleterious effects on fertility. Furthermore, couples in which the male partner has diabetes mellitus have a significantly longer time to pregnancy.[5,6] Depending on the endocrinopathy, infertility can be reversible or potentially indicative of significant medical pathology.[1,7]

Endocrine regulation of spermatogenesis and testicular function is dependent on an intact hypothalamic-pituitary-testicular axis (**Fig. 1**). The hypothalamus produces and secretes gonadotropin-releasing hormone (GnRH), which is carried through the portal circulation to the pituitary gland. In response to GnRH, the gonadotropic cells of the anterior pituitary secrete luteinizing hormone (LH) and follicle-stimulating hormone (FSH). These hormones circulate systemically and bind to membrane receptors on target organs. LH stimulates the production of sex steroids in the Leydig cells of the testicle. FSH supports the function of the Sertoli cells in the seminiferous tubules, which are critical for sperm cell maturation. The Leydig cells mainly generate testosterone, which is secreted in a pulsatile manner and binds to serum proteins like albumin and sex hormone–binding globulin (SHBG). Leydig cells also produce smaller amounts of estradiol and dihydrotestosterone. However, the main source of estradiol in the body is the peripheral conversion of testosterone via aromatase in adipose tissues. Dihydrotestosterone is also produced in other organs like the

[a] Baylor College of Medicine, 1 Baylor Plaza, Houston, TX 77030, USA; [b] Division of Urology, Department of Surgery, University of Utah School of Medicine, 3 North 1900 East, Salt Lake City, UT 84132, USA
* Corresponding author.
E-mail address: alexander.pastuszak@hsc.utah.edu

Urol Clin N Am 47 (2020) 139–146
https://doi.org/10.1016/j.ucl.2019.12.002

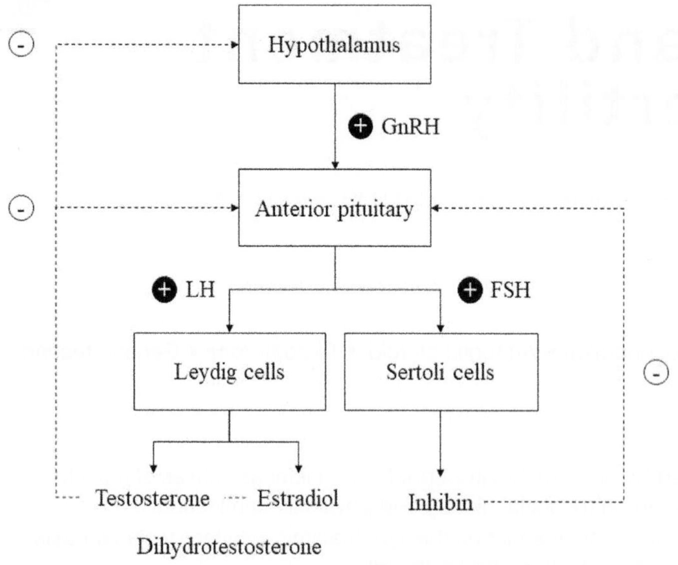

Fig. 1. The hypothalamic-pituitary-testicular axis with end products that regulate feedback inhibition.

prostate and epididymis, which contain 5-alpha-reductase for the conversion of testosterone. Regulation of gonadotropic cell products LH and FSH is maintained by feedback inhibition from the production of testosterone, estradiol, and inhibin, a regulatory hormone produced and released by the Sertoli cells.

The design of the hypothalamic-pituitary-testicular axis is elegant but can result in aberrant hormone signaling when there is a defect at any point along the pathway. Furthermore, exogenous administration of end products can result in dysfunction in an otherwise intact endocrine system. For example, exogenous testosterone does not directly affect the intratesticular concentration of testosterone because of the tight junctions in the blood-testicular barrier. However, the serum level of testosterone rises with supplementation and inhibits the production of LH and FSH, resulting in a paradoxic decrease in intratesticular testosterone production.[8] The endocrinopathies that disrupt male fertility can be grouped into categories, such as hypothalamic disease, pituitary disease, primary and secondary hypogonadism, and other pre-testicular causes[9–12] (**Table 1**).

EVALUATION

Due to the wide range of endocrinopathies, health care practitioners must have a systematic approach. Before considering endocrine etiologies for male factor infertility, an initial evaluation must be completed. This is typically performed in the outpatient setting and begins with a complete history, with careful attention to the reproductive and sexual history. This consists of the following:

- Coital frequency, timing, and use of lubricants
- Prior history of pregnancies for either the male or female partner
- Erectile and ejaculatory function
- Duration of infertility and prior fertility
- Childhood illnesses and development
- History of urologic trauma or disease (eg, epididymitis, orchitis, sexually transmitted infection)
- Past medical and surgical history
- Medications and supplements
- Family history of infertility
- History of traumatic brain injury
- Exposure to wet heat, chemicals, toxins, drugs, or radiation

When reviewing medications, physicians must also specifically ask about prior or present testosterone and/or anabolic steroid use. Careful evaluation of dietary and nutritional supplement usage is critical, as their ingredients are not regulated by the Food and Drug Administration (FDA). Studies have demonstrated that more than 20% of legally sold supplements contain anabolic steroids not listed on nutritional labels.[13–15]

The initial evaluation also includes a comprehensive physical examination and 2 semen analyses. Urologists should perform a thorough genitourinary examination in addition to noting body habitus, development of age-appropriate male secondary sex characteristics, and presence of any signs that could suggest an underlying

Table 1
Table of endocrine-related disorders that can result in male factor infertility

Hypothalamic	Testicular
Tumors, for example, craniopharyngioma, secondary metastasis	Anorchia, for example, viral orchitis, testicular torsion
Infiltrative disease, for example, tuberculosis, sarcoidosis	Other causes
	Klinefelter syndrome
Cranial radiation	Diabetes mellitus
Pituitary	Obesity
Tumors, for example, prolactinoma	Thyroid disease
Acromegaly	Congenital adrenal hyperplasia
Cushing disease	Androgen resistance
Hyperprolactinemia	Exogenous androgen administration
Kallmann syndrome	Illicit drugs, for example, anabolic steroids, cannabis
Empty sella syndrome	
Pituitary stalk interruption syndrome	Eating disorders
Pituitary stalk transection, for example, trauma	Medications

endocrinopathy (eg, gynecomastia, striae, thyroid enlargement). Multiple international guidelines recommend 2 semen analyses separated by at least 1 month if possible.[1,16–19] Although a single semen sample cannot be relied on to exclude abnormal spermatogenesis, the presence of multiple severe semen parameter abnormalities may obviate the need for a second semen analysis, as it would not significantly alter management and would otherwise delay treatment.[20]

Absolute indications for endocrine evaluation include an abnormal semen analysis, impaired sexual function, or clinical findings in the history or physical examination suggestive of a specific endocrinopathy.[21] There is ongoing debate as to whether all men presenting for fertility evaluation should undergo an endocrine evaluation. Studies that support evaluation of hormone levels during the initial evaluation associate low total serum testosterone with abnormal sperm morphology and lower live birth rates.[22,23] Patel and colleagues[24] also found low total serum testosterone in men with idiopathic infertility and normal sperm concentrations, which would have been missed had a hormonal evaluation not been performed. On the other hand, endocrine causes of male factor infertility are uncommon. Although the individual cost of a blood draw and serum hormone analysis is relatively affordable, the annual cost to the medical system is greater and may be as high as $70,000.[2] The American Society for Reproductive Medicine acknowledges that there is no consensus, but it is the opinion of this expert that hormonal evaluation should be performed at the initial evaluation of the infertile male.

An endocrine evaluation for infertility should at minimum consist of serum testosterone and FSH levels.[21] Most infertility experts additionally measure serum levels of free testosterone, sex hormone–binding globulin, prolactin, and LH. Although serum inhibin B is superior to FSH as a marker of spermatogenesis, FSH remains the preferred screening test in practice because of the high cost of serum inhibin B analysis.[25] Physicians also should consider estradiol and thyroid function studies, as alterations in these hormones can have a negative effect on sexual function and fertility.[12] Imaging also may be warranted as part of the endocrine evaluation if there are abnormal laboratory results (eg, brain MRI for elevated prolactin).

TREATMENT

The goal of treatment is to correct any reversible hormonal pathology and restore fertility. If restoration of fertility is not possible, then it is important for urologists to counsel the couple on prognosis, as this can provide relief and an opportunity to recommend other methods of parenthood (eg, adoption). The remainder of this section addresses the current research and standards of care for endocrinopathies that impact function of the hypothalamic-pituitary-testicular axis.

HYPERGONADOTROPIC HYPOGONADISM

Primary hypogonadism, also known as hypergonadotropic hypogonadism or primary testicular failure, is diagnosed via the presence of low testosterone despite high levels of GnRH, LH, and FSH. The pathology underlying this hypergonadotropic state can be congenital or acquired.

Klinefelter syndrome is the most common congenital etiology of hypergonadotropic hypogonadism, as well as the most common sex chromosome disorder overall, affecting approximately 1 in 500 male individuals.[26] It is characterized by aneuploidy of the sex chromosomes, with most cases displaying a 47, XXY genotype. Clinical findings include above-average height, eunuchoid body habitus, gynecomastia, and small testes. However, these symptoms can be subtle and the initial presentation for these men can occur during adulthood as difficulty with conception. Diagnosis is established by karyotyping, although a normal karyotype can be present in up to 20% of men with mosaic Klinefelter syndrome.[27] Although men with Klinefelter syndrome were previously thought to be irreversibly sterile, use of conventional testicular sperm extraction (TESE) or microsurgical TESE (microTESE) with intracytoplasmic sperm injection has allowed some to achieve pregnancy with their partners. Literature suggests that urologists should discuss family planning with these men early, as extraction of viable sperm is less successful with older age.[28] Some experts also have called for studies examining the success of TESE in adolescents with Klinefelter syndrome, as significantly more sperm may be retrieved for cryopreservation before the initiation of hormone therapy for secondary sexual characteristics.[29]

Variants in the genes associated with the beta subunit of gonadotropins and their associated receptors also have been linked to primary testicular failure.[30–34] Acquired etiologies of hypergonadotropic hypogonadism are typically caused by direct testicular insult and include anorchia, testicular torsion or trauma, viral orchitis, chemotherapeutic toxins, and radiation. These conditions are generally irreversible, and options for future fertility are limited to surgical retrieval of sperm or donor insemination.

HYPOGONADOTROPIC HYPOGONADISM

Secondary hypogonadism is characterized by low testosterone in the presence of low GnRH, LH, and FSH levels. This clinical presentation is also referred to in the literature as hypogonadotropic hypogonadism or secondary testicular failure. In patients with acquired secondary hypogonadism, evaluation with thyroid and adrenal function studies, serum prolactin, and cranial MRI should be performed to rule out structural abnormalities of the pituitary (eg, prolactinoma).

Current literature has suggested that anabolic steroid–induced hypogonadism is now the most common cause of hypogonadism among men.[35] Anabolic steroid use is a growing public health concern, as these substances are increasingly used by younger men of reproductive age, with a lifetime prevalence use of 3% to 4%.[36,37] The mechanism by which anabolic steroids result in hypogonadotropic hypogonadism is via inhibition of GnRH release through a negative feedback loop, ultimately decreasing signaling for intratesticular production of testosterone. Although these drugs may have the desired effect of increased muscle mass, their androgenic component commonly produces side effects of gynecomastia, testicular atrophy, sexual dysfunction, and infertility secondary to decreased spermatogenesis, among others.[37] All patients should be counseled to discontinue anabolic steroid use in the interest of fertility and overall health.[9,38] After suspending use, the literature suggests that average time to recovery of spermatogenesis (>5 million sperm per milliliter) ranges from 4 to 12 months.[39,40] If spermatogenesis does not return after 4 months, then it is possible these patients had underlying, undiagnosed infertility and urologists should consider alternate diagnostic evaluations.[41]

Exogenous testosterone administration can result in infertility due to a paradoxic decrease in intratesticular testosterone levels via the same mechanism by which anabolic steroids inhibit testosterone production. Although prescribing of testosterone is decreasing nationally (eg, 40% decline within the Veterans Administration system), testosterone prescriptions in America surged from 1.2 million in 2010 to 2.2 million in 2013.[42–44] A survey of American Urologic Association urologists found that approximately 25% have prescribed testosterone for infertility associated with low testosterone.[45] Outcomes are generally favorable after discontinuation of testosterone, but risk factors for prolonged infertility include increased duration of exogenous testosterone use and older age, independent of puberty.[34,40]

If patients with prior anabolic steroid or testosterone use are persistently hypogonadal after discontinuation, then pharmacologic management can be considered. Some experts suggest implementing medical therapy early, for example, when anabolic steroids are discontinued.[46] Clomiphene citrate, a selective estrogen receptor modulator (SERM) that prevents the inhibitory effects of estrogen on LH and FSH, is often used initially, as it is relatively inexpensive, available in an oral formulation, and has been demonstrated as safe and efficacious for long-term use.[47] In this expert's experience, the combined use of clomiphene citrate and human chorionic gonadotropin (HCG) provides a rapid return to spermatogenesis. The adjunct use of FSH in addition to the preceding pharmacologic therapies can be considered in men who are refractory to clomiphene and HCG. Notably, the use of clomiphene may be limited by estrogenic effects, limiting its benefit.[48]

In select patients with testosterone-to-estradiol ratios of less than 10:1, aromatase inhibitors can be used to decrease estrogen production.[49] This class of medications achieves the same effect as SERMs by decreasing estrogen feedback to the pituitary, resulting in increased testosterone production and spermatogenesis. However, long-term use of aromatase inhibitors is associated with osteoporosis in women, although the long-term effects in men are uncertain.

HCG mimics LH function with a structurally similar beta subunit. HCG is the only FDA-approved treatment for secondary hypogonadism, although studies on its safety with long-term use are lacking. Even with concurrent testosterone therapy, HCG can maintain spermatogenesis relatively well and can be prescribed as concurrent therapy with testosterone.[50,51] All medications other than testosterone that are currently used for the treatment of hypogonadotropic hypogonadism are considered off-label, and patients should be appropriately counseled on potential risks. HCG-based therapy in combination with SERMs, aromatase inhibitors, or recombinant FSH is a promising treatment for testosterone-related infertility, with an improvement in spermatogenesis observed in approximately 96% of participants.[51] However, a limitation of this study, as with most of the literature on this topic, is the lack of a control group to mitigate temporal treatment bias. Superiority of medication to discontinuation alone has not yet been demonstrated in the literature and requires further investigation.

Other acquired forms of secondary hypogonadism include hypothalamic and pituitary disorders. Pituitary adenomas are the most common pituitary pathology.[52] Of these, functioning tumors such as prolactinomas occur more often in young adults of reproductive age. Excess prolactin can result in galactorrhea and bitemporal hemianopsia. Medical management with dopamine agonists is sufficient for most patients with prolactinomas, as these tumors rarely require surgery or radiation. Gonadotropin deficiency also can result from head trauma through damage to the pituitary (eg, transection of the pituitary stalk). Patients with history of traumatic brain injury should be monitored for the development of gonadotropin deficiency, as a prospective study demonstrated the prevalence of hypogonadism to be 7.7% at 12-month follow-up.[53] Insults to the hypothalamus also can result in secondary hypogonadism. Although not as well studied in men as compared with women, eating disorders in men appear to have similar suppression of the hypothalamus that can result in decreased GnRH release.[11] Conversely, diabetes mellitus and obesity result in an excess estrogen state that suppresses the release of gonadotropins and can result in infertility. Infiltrative diseases like sarcoidosis also can present with hypothalamic-pituitary disease that results in clinically significant hypogonadism.[54]

Congenital hypogonadotropic hypogonadism results from impaired migration of GnRH-producing neurons. Patients with this condition can present with impaired sense of smell, which is referred to as Kallmann syndrome, and occurs from simultaneous failure of olfactory neuron migration. Other signs of congenital hypogonadotropic hypogonadism include unilateral renal agenesis, absence of secondary sexual characteristics, and cryptorchidism, the last of which prognosticates a poor response to fertility therapy.[55] Although patients with congenital hypogonadotropic hypogonadism were previously accepted as infertile, reversal of secondary testicular failure has been demonstrated in up to 20% of them.[56,57] Treatment options directed at fertility include pump-administered pulsatile GnRH or subcutaneous gonadotropin injections. However, there is limited evidence for comparing efficacy in stimulating spermatogenesis. Most men with congenital hypogonadotropic hypogonadism rarely achieve normal sperm counts, but fertility is attainable with reports of successful pregnancies after hormonal therapy.[58,59]

FUTURE DIRECTIONS

As we better understand the genetic basis of male infertility, future male factor infertility evaluations will likely include routine genetic screening. Currently, guidelines recommend genetic screening for men with azoospermia or severe oligospermia.[16] Available technologies in clinical practice can screen for autosomal gene variants (eg, CFTR in cystic fibrosis), chromosomal abnormalities, and Y chromosome microdeletions, which are all gene factors that have been shown to impact male fertility. Use of newer methods, like microarray analysis and whole-genome sequencing, have yielded candidate genes that are related to endocrine function in infertile men, but are not in broad clinical use yet (**Table 2**).

In the context of precision medicine, genetic testing also may guide treatment selection for men with male infertility. The best example of this currently in the literature is selection of patients for pharmacologic therapy with FSH. Research has demonstrated that polymorphisms in FSH receptor genes are associated with significant difference in semen parameters after FSH treatment.[60] In addition, polymorphisms in the FSH beta subunit also may have clinical significance. Studies

Table 2
Endocrine disorder–linked genes that may result in male factor infertility

Abnormal hypothalamus development and function	Adrenal gland dysfunction
ANOS1	CYP11A1
CHD7	CYP11B1
FGFR1	CYP17A1
KISS1R	CYP19A1
PROKR2	CYP21A2
TACR3	NROB1
FGF8	HSD3B2
PLXNA1	Abnormal development of reproductive organs
PROK2	AMH
SOX2	AMHR
SOX10	AR
WDR11	NR5A1
CCDC141	SRD5A2
DCC	SRY
GHRH1	WT1
HS6ST1	MAMLD1
SEMA3A	SOX3
Pituitary gland dysfunction	GATA4
GNRHR	HSD17B3
LHB	SOX9
FSHB	RSPO1
FSHR	

Adapted from Ferlin A, Dipresa S, Delbarba A, et al. Contemporary genetics-based diagnostics of male infertility. Expert Rev Mol Diagn. 2019;19(7):623–633. doi:10.1080/14737159.2019.1633917.

by Grigorova and colleagues[61,62] examined men with variants in the −211 base pair promotor regions for the FSH beta subunit and found that these men have lower serum levels of FSH. Larger studies are warranted to determine the clinical utility of candidate genes, although approximately 1200 to 1500 genes linked to male infertility have been identified to date.

One current barrier to genetic testing is cost. On average, whole-genome sequencing costs approximately $1000. In a national survey, more than half of the respondents would not pay more than $500 for actionable sequencing and more than a third would not pay more than $200.[63] Fortunately, trends have shown that cost is decreasing with time. Future developments in technology may eventually make advanced genetic analysis techniques affordable and available to even the most socioeconomically disadvantaged patients.

SUMMARY

Endocrinopathies are rare causes of male factor infertility but should be considered in all evaluations because of their prognosis for infertility and overall health. Diagnosis of an endocrine-related infertility can potentially save couples from undergoing the stress of an expensive artificial insemination process. Optimal evaluation of endocrine disorders is systematic, and includes a thorough history, physical examination, and semen analysis. Most infertility experts would agree that serum hormone laboratories should be included in the initial infertility evaluation, as they are relatively inexpensive. Treatment is dependent on the endocrine disorder, but advances in genetic testing could further assist in determining patient responsiveness to pharmacologic therapies.

DISCLOSURE

The authors have nothing to disclose.

REFERENCES

1. Honig SC, Lipshultz LI, Jarow J. Significant medical pathology uncovered by a comprehensive male infertility evaluation. Fertil Steril 1994;62(5):1028–34. Available at: http://www.ncbi.nlm.nih.gov/pubmed/7926114. Accessed September 9, 2019.
2. Sigman M, Jarow JP. Endocrine evaluation of infertile men. Urology 1997;50(5):659–64.
3. Esteves SC, Miyaoka R, Agarwal A. An update on the clinical assessment of the infertile male. Clinics (Sau Paulo) 2011;66(4):691–700.
4. Krausz C. Male infertility: pathogenesis and clinical diagnosis. Best Pract Res Clin Endocrinol Metab 2011;25(2):271–85.
5. Kasturi SS, Tannir J, Brannigan RE. The metabolic syndrome and male infertility. J Androl 2008;29(3):251–9.
6. Eisenberg ML, Sundaram R, Maisog J, et al. Diabetes, medical comorbidities and couple fecundity. Hum Reprod 2016;31(10):2369–76.
7. Kolettis PN, Sabanegh ES. Significant medical pathology discovered during a male infertility evaluation. J Urol 2001;166(1):178–80. Available at: http://www.ncbi.nlm.nih.gov/pubmed/11435851. Accessed September 9, 2019.
8. Jarow JP, Chen H, Rosner W, et al. Assessment of the androgen environment within the human testis: minimally invasive method to obtain intratesticular fluid. J Androl 2001;22(4):640–5.
9. Jarow JP, Lipshultz LI. Anabolic steroid-induced hypogonadotropic hypogonadism. Am J Sports Med 1990;18(4):429–31.
10. Bellis MA, Hughes K, Calafat A, et al. Sexual uses of alcohol and drugs and the associated health risks: a cross sectional study of young people in nine European cities. BMC Public Health 2008;8:155.

11. Skolnick A, Schulman RC, Galindo RJ, et al. The endocrinopathies of male anorexia nervosa: a case series. AACE Clin Case Rep 2016;2(4):e351–7.
12. Bates JN, Kohn TP, Pastuszak AW. Effect of thyroid hormone derangements on sexual function in men and women. Sex Med Rev 2018. https://doi.org/10.1016/j.sxmr.2018.09.005.
13. Geyer H, Parr MK, Mareck U, et al. Analysis of non-hormonal nutritional supplements for anabolic-androgenic steroids - results of an international study. Int J Sports Med 2004;25(2):124–9.
14. Geyer H, Parr MK, Koehler K, et al. Nutritional supplements cross-contaminated and faked with doping substances. J Mass Spectrom 2008;43(7):892–902.
15. Baume N, Mahler N, Kamber M, et al. Research of stimulants and anabolic steroids in dietary supplements. Scand J Med Sci Sports 2006;16(1):41–8.
16. Jarow J, Sigman M, Kolettis PN, et al. Optimal evaluation of the infertile male - American Urological Association. AUA Best Practice. Available at: https://www.auanet.org/guidelines/male-infertility-optimal-evaluation-best-practice-statement. Accessed September 8, 2019.
17. World Health Organization. WHO laboratory manual for the examination and processing of human semen. 5th ed. Geneva: WHO Press; 2010.
18. Blickenstorfer K, Voelkle M, Xie M, et al. Are WHO recommendations to perform 2 consecutive semen analyses for reliable diagnosis of male infertility still valid? J Urol 2019;201(4):783–91.
19. Nagler HM. Male factor infertility: a solitary semen analysis can never predict normal fertility. Nat Rev Urol 2011;8(1):16–7.
20. Keihani S, Pastuszak AW, Hotaling JM. Re: are WHO recommendations to perform 2 consecutive semen analyses for reliable diagnosis of male infertility still valid? J Urol 2019. https://doi.org/10.1097/JU.0000000000000413.
21. Pfeifer S, Butts S, Dumesic D, et al. Diagnostic evaluation of the infertile male: a committee opinion. Fertil Steril 2015;103(3):e18–25.
22. Trussell JC, Coward RM, Santoro N, et al. Association between testosterone, semen parameters, and live birth in men with unexplained infertility in an intrauterine insemination population. Fertil Steril 2019;111(6):1129–34.
23. Mumford SL, Hotaling JM. Should all men being evaluated for couple infertility have an endocrine and reproductive urology evaluation? Fertil Steril 2019;111(6):1107–8.
24. Patel DP, Brant WO, Myers JB, et al. Sperm concentration is poorly associated with hypoandrogenism in infertile men. Urology 2015;85(5):1062–7.
25. Kumanov P, Nandipati K, Tomova A, et al. Inhibin B is a better marker of spermatogenesis than other hormones in the evaluation of male factor infertility. Fertil Steril 2006;86(2):332–8.
26. Bojesen A, Juul S, Gravholt CH. Prenatal and postnatal prevalence of Klinefelter syndrome: a national registry study. J Clin Endocrinol Metab 2003;88(2):622–6.
27. Abdelmoula NB, Amouri A, Portnoi MF, et al. Cytogenetics and fluorescence in situ hybridization assessment of sex-chromosome mosaicism in Klinefelter's syndrome. Ann Genet 2004;47(2):163–75.
28. Okada H, Goda K, Yamamoto Y, et al. Age as a limiting factor for successful sperm retrieval in patients with nonmosaic Klinefelter's syndrome. Fertil Steril 2005;84(6):1662–4.
29. Lejeune H, Brosse A, Groupe Fertipreserve, Plotton I. Fertility in Klinefelter syndrome. Presse Med 2014;43(2):162–70.
30. Lindstedt G, Nyström E, Matthews C, et al. Follitropin (FSH) deficiency in an infertile male due to FSHbeta gene mutation. A syndrome of normal puberty and virilization but underdeveloped testicles with azoospermia, low FSH but high lutropin and normal serum testosterone concentrations. Clin Chem Lab Med 1998;36(8):663–5.
31. Latronico AC, Anasti J, Arnhold IJ, et al. Brief report: testicular and ovarian resistance to luteinizing hormone caused by inactivating mutations of the luteinizing hormone-receptor gene. N Engl J Med 1996;334(8):507–12.
32. Kremer H, Kraaij R, Toledo SP, et al. Male pseudohermaphroditism due to a homozygous missense mutation of the luteinizing hormone receptor gene. Nat Genet 1995;9(2):160–4.
33. Weiss J, Axelrod L, Whitcomb RW, et al. Hypogonadism caused by a single amino acid substitution in the beta subunit of luteinizing hormone. N Engl J Med 1992;326(3):179–83.
34. Hendriks AEJ, Boellaard WPA, Van Casteren NJ, et al. Fatherhood in tall men treated with high-dose sex steroids during adolescence. J Clin Endocrinol Metab 2010;95(12):5233–40.
35. Coward RM, Rajanahally S, Kovac JR, et al. Anabolic steroid induced hypogonadism in young men. J Urol 2013;190(6):2200–5.
36. Sjöqvist F, Garle M, Rane A. Use of doping agents, particularly anabolic steroids, in sports and society. Lancet 2008;371(9627):1872–82.
37. Fronczak CM, Kim ED, Barqawi AB. The insults of illicit drug use on male fertility. J Androl 2012;33(4):515–28.
38. Knuth UA, Maniera H, Nieschlag E. Anabolic steroids and semen parameters in bodybuilders. Fertil Steril 1989;52(6):1041–7.
39. de Souza GL, Hallak J. Anabolic steroids and male infertility: a comprehensive review. BJU Int 2011;108(11):1860–5.

40. Kohn TP, Louis MR, Pickett SM, et al. Age and duration of testosterone therapy predict time to return of sperm count after human chorionic gonadotropin therapy. Fertil Steril 2017;107(2):351–7.e1.
41. Nieschlag E, Vorona E. Medical consequences of doping with anabolic androgenic steroids: effects on reproductive functions. Eur J Endocrinol 2015; 173(2):R47–58.
42. Baillargeon J, Kuo YF, Westra JR, et al. Testosterone prescribing in the United States, 2002-2016. J Am Med Assoc 2018;320(2):200–2.
43. Nguyen CP, Hirsch MS, Moeny D, et al. Testosterone and "age-related hypogonadism" - FDA concerns. N Engl J Med 2015;373(8):689–91.
44. Jasuja GK, Bhasin S, Rose AJ. Patterns of testosterone prescription overuse. Curr Opin Endocrinol Diabetes Obes 2017;24(3):240–5.
45. Ko EY, Siddiqi K, Brannigan RE, et al. Empirical medical therapy for idiopathic male infertility: a survey of the American Urological Association. J Urol 2012;187(3):973–8.
46. Rahnema CD, Lipshultz LI, Crosnoe LE, et al. Anabolic steroid-induced hypogonadism: diagnosis and treatment. Fertil Steril 2014;101(5):1271–9.
47. Moskovic DJ, Katz DJ, Akhavan A, et al. Clomiphene citrate is safe and effective for long-term management of hypogonadism. BJU Int 2012;110(10): 1524–8.
48. Hussein A, Ozgok Y, Ross L, et al. Optimization of spermatogenesis-regulating hormones in patients with non-obstructive azoospermia and its impact on sperm retrieval: a multicentre study. BJU Int 2013;111(3 Pt B):E110–4.
49. Raman JD, Schlegel PN. Aromatase inhibitors for male infertility. J Urol 2002;167(2 Pt 1):624–9.
50. Hsieh T-C, Pastuszak AW, Hwang K, et al. Concomitant intramuscular human chorionic gonadotropin preserves spermatogenesis in men undergoing testosterone replacement therapy. J Urol 2013; 189(2):647–50.
51. Wenker EP, Dupree JM, Langille GM, et al. The use of HCG-based combination therapy for recovery of spermatogenesis after testosterone use. J Sex Med 2015;12(6):1334–7.
52. Famini P, Maya MM, Melmed S. Pituitary magnetic resonance imaging for sellar and parasellar masses: ten-year experience in 2598 patients. J Clin Endocrinol Metab 2011;96(6):1633–41.
53. Tanriverdi F, Senyurek H, Unluhizarci K, et al. High risk of hypopituitarism after traumatic brain injury: a prospective investigation of anterior pituitary function in the acute phase and 12 months after trauma. J Clin Endocrinol Metab 2006;91(6):2105–11.
54. Bihan H, Christozova V, Dumas JL, et al. Sarcoidosis: clinical, hormonal, and magnetic resonance imaging (MRI) manifestations of hypothalamic-pituitary disease in 9 patients and review of the literature. Medicine (Baltimore) 2007;86(5):259–68.
55. Miyagawa Y, Tsujimura A, Matsumiya K, et al. Outcome of gonadotropin therapy for male hypogonadotropic hypogonadism at university affiliated male infertility centers: a 30-year retrospective study. J Urol 2005;173(6):2072–5.
56. Raivio T, Falardeau J, Dwyer A, et al. Reversal of idiopathic hypogonadotropic hypogonadism. N Engl J Med 2007;357(9):863–73.
57. Sidhoum VF, Chan YM, Lippincott MF, et al. Reversal and relapse of hypogonadotropic hypogonadism: resilience and fragility of the reproductive neuroendocrine system. J Clin Endocrinol Metab 2014; 99(3):861–70.
58. Rastrelli G, Corona G, Mannucci E, et al. Factors affecting spermatogenesis upon gonadotropin-replacement therapy: a meta-analytic study. Andrology 2014;2(6):794–808.
59. Boehm U, Bouloux PM, Dattani MT, et al. Expert consensus document: European Consensus Statement on congenital hypogonadotropic hypogonadism–pathogenesis, diagnosis and treatment. Nat Rev Endocrinol 2015;11(9):547–64.
60. Simoni M, Santi D, Negri L, et al. Treatment with human, recombinant FSH improves sperm DNA fragmentation in idiopathic infertile men depending on the FSH receptor polymorphism p.N680S: a pharmacogenetic study. Hum Reprod 2016;31(9): 1960–9.
61. Grigorova M, Punab M, Poolamets O, et al. Increased prevalance of the -211 T allele of follicle stimulating hormone (FSH) beta subunit promoter polymorphism and lower serum FSH in infertile men. J Clin Endocrinol Metab 2010;95(1):100–8.
62. Grigorova M, Punab M, Ausmees K, et al. FSHB promoter polymorphism within evolutionary conserved element is associated with serum FSH level in men. Hum Reprod 2008;23(9):2160–6.
63. Marshall DA, Gonzalez JM, Johnson FR, et al. What are people willing to pay for whole-genome sequencing information, and who decides what they receive? Genet Med 2016;18(12):1295–302.

Sperm Extraction in Obstructive Azoospermia

What's Next?

Jason P. Akerman, MD, FRCSC[a,*], Solomon Hayon, MD[a], Robert Matthew Coward, MD, FACS[a,b]

KEYWORDS

• Sperm retrieval • Obstructive azoospermia • Infertility

KEY POINTS

- The evolution of operative techniques for sperm retrieval, coupled with the introduction of in vitro fertilization and intracytoplasmic sperm injection, have afforded previously untreatable men with obstructive azoospermia reliable pathways to conception.
- Percutaneous sperm aspiration techniques have remained highly effective tools with minimal modifications since their introduction.
- Open approaches to sperm extraction continue to shift toward more minimally invasive practices in the hopes of facilitating their use in the clinic setting while minimizing patient morbidity.
- Innovations in sperm selection and purification may offer a means of improving the fertility potential of specimens and address important sperm parameters, including DNA fragmentation.

INTRODUCTION

Advancements in operative technology, coupled with the introduction of in vitro fertilization (IVF) and intracytoplasmic sperm injection (ICSI), have afforded previously untreatable infertile men with reliable pathways to conception. In particular, the introduction of the surgical microscope revolutionized the surgical management of male infertility and sperm retrieval. For men with obstructive azoospermia (OA), sperm can now be extracted from several different sites using a variety of surgical techniques. The obstruction can occur anywhere along the passage of sperm from the efferent ducts within the testis, along the epididymis, through the vas deferens, the ejaculatory ducts, the penile urethra, or even the urethral meatus. Of the 15% of infertile men presenting with azoospermia, approximately 30% to 40% have an obstructive cause.[1,2] Because of preserved spermatogenesis, sperm extraction with high-quality samples can be obtained upstream from the site of obstruction or by relieving the obstruction itself. This extraction is accomplished through reconstructive microsurgery, resection of the obstruction, percutaneous aspiration, or open surgical retrieval.

Although the last few decades have produced reliable surgical options for men with OA, further advances show promise in improving outcomes, reducing surgical time, and decreasing procedure-related morbidity. This article traces the evolution of sperm extraction techniques for OA and highlights new developments and innovations in sperm selection and purification.

HISTORY AND EVOLUTION OF SPERM EXTRACTION TECHNIQUES

The first reported use of aspirated sperm was published by Temple-Smith and colleagues[3] in 1985. The case involved a 42-year-old man with a history

[a] Department of Urology, University of North Carolina, 2113 Physician's Office Building, CB#7235, Chapel Hill, NC 27599-7235, USA; [b] UNC Fertility, 7920 ACC Blvd #300, Raleigh, North Carolina 27617, USA
* Corresponding author.
E-mail address: Jason.akerman@med.unc.edu

Urol Clin N Am 47 (2020) 147–155
https://doi.org/10.1016/j.ucl.2019.12.003

of vasectomy and 2 subsequent failed reversals with vasoepididymostomy. Following prolonged epididymal massage and aspiration, a total of 0.2 mL was retrieved with 76% motility and an estimated concentration of 4.28×10^6 sperm per milliliter. Successful fertilization and clinical pregnancy was achieved through IVF using this sample. Building on this work, Silber and colleagues[4] published their approach to microsurgical epididymal sperm aspiration (MESA) in 1988. The article outlines a technique for epididymal sperm aspiration under 10 to 40 times magnification that begins in the distal corpus of the epididymis and continues proximally until motile sperm are retrieved. The 2 patients in whom this procedure was initially described both had congenital bilateral absence of the vas deferens (CBAVD). This new technique to be used in conjunction with IVF was well received and offered a path to pregnancy for men with OA. However, early fertilization and pregnancy rates did not produce favorable results. Many centers reported a success rate less than 10%.[5] Poor fertilization and pregnancy rates, coupled with the need for an operative microscope, limited the initial uptake of the MESA approach. The advent of ICSI a few years later led to significant improvements in outcomes with epididymal sperm.[5] With these changes came renewed interest in MESA. More recently, modifications to the MESA technique have been published, including the mini-MESA, obliterative MESA, and minimally invasive epididymal sperm aspiration (MIESA).[6–8]

Nearly 10 years after Temple-Smith and colleagues[3] published their technique of epididymal sperm aspiration, Craft and colleagues[9] described a percutaneous approach using a 21-gauge needle. This approach formed the basis of what is now considered a conventional percutaneous epididymal sperm aspiration (PESA). The procedure was well received because many surgeons did not have access to an operating microscope to perform MESA. PESA was initially performed with intravenous or general anesthesia but is now commonly done with local anesthesia in the office setting.[7]

The introduction of ICSI in 1992 made it possible to use sperm aspirated from the testes.[10] The first uses of testicular sperm for fertilization were reported in 1993 by Schoysman and colleagues.[11] They describe obtaining samples by testicular biopsy in men who were previously unable to produce an epididymal sperm sample. This technique is now commonly referred to as testicular sperm extraction (TESE). Using ICSI, successful fertilization and pregnancy was achieved.[11] This method overcame initial concerns of the fertilizing potential of less mature testicular sperm. In an attempt to minimize morbidity, percutaneous testicular sperm aspiration (TESA) was explored. Before this, TESA had been described as a diagnostic tool in azoospermic men.[12] The first report of TESA for ICSI was published by Bourne and colleagues[13] in 1995. Their technique used a 20-gauge Menghini biopsy needle under negative pressure in 2 men with OA. High rates of normal fertilization and subsequent pregnancy were achieved using the aspirated sample.[13] TESA was seen as a way to overcome the need for an operative microscope, avoid general anesthesia, and reduce patient morbidity. The procedure has evolved over time to include multiple needle passes with thinner-gauge needles.[12–15] The most recent development in sperm retrieval from the testis is microdissection testicular sperm extraction as first described by Peter Schlegel[16] in 1999. After observing that seminiferous tubules had different morphologic characteristics under the operating microscope, selective extraction of larger tubules (more likely to contain sperm) was performed. This technique allowed improved identification and retrieval of sperm while removing less tissue from the testis. For men with nonobstructive azoospermia (NOA), the technique has emerged as a more effective and reliable technique than multiple-pass TESE.[10]

Given the success of TESA and PESA percutaneous approaches, Qiu and colleagues[17] explored vasal sperm aspiration as another means of obtaining sperm percutaneously. Their 1997 article discussed percutaneous vasal sperm aspiration (PVSA) in 6 men diagnosed with ejaculatory duct obstruction. Of the 6 men included in the study, adequate sperm for intrauterine insemination (IUI) was obtained in 3 men. Only 1 resulted in a pregnancy. With the vas deferens fixed to the skin by a clip, a 21-gauge needle was advanced into the lumen of the vas deferens followed by a 23-gauge blunt needle. The 23-gauge needle was advanced through the 21-gauge needle in the direction of the epididymis. Aspiration was done using a 5-mL syringe.[17] The evolution of sperm retrieval techniques is shown in **Fig. 1**.

CURRENT ROLE OF EPIDIDYMAL AND TESTICULAR SPERM RETRIEVAL IN OBSTRUCTIVE AZOOSPERMIA

Percutaneous Approaches to Sperm Retrieval

Percutaneous methods of sperm retrieval provide several benefits to both patients and surgeons. These procedures are particularly appealing because they can be performed on short notice under local anesthesia in the outpatient setting,

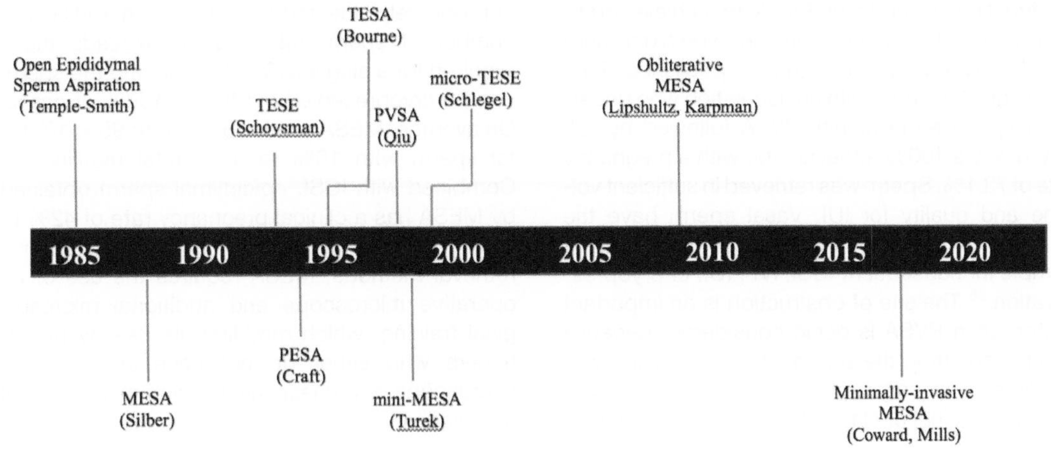

Fig. 1. Timeline of sperm retrieval techniques.

have minimal patient downtime, and are highly reproducible. Unlike more invasive methods of sperm retrieval, percutaneous aspiration does not require additional equipment or training in microsurgery. Percutaneous sperm extraction can be targeted at the level of the testis, epididymis, or vas deferens.

Percutaneous Epididymal Sperm Aspiration

Among men with OA, sperm retrieval rates with PESA range from 51% to 100%, irrespective of the cause of their obstruction.[7] Retrieval of motile sperm is high, with reported rates ranging from 62% to 94%.[18] In men with postvasectomy OA who do not desire a reversal, PESA offers an appealing method of sperm extraction. Collins and colleagues[19] reported one of the few comparative studies with PESA as an intervention. They performed MESA and PESA on both testes in men with previously proven fertility seeking vasectomy reversal. There was no difference in the rate of successful sperm retrieval between MESA and PESA. These investigators therefore advocate PESA when possible in men with OA secondary to vasectomy. More recently, Yafi and Zini[18] reported on 255 men with OA undergoing PESA. The study included men with OA of various causes, including vasectomy, vasectomy with prior failed reversal, and CBAVD. Motile sperm was found in 75.3% of men. Younger paternal age and testicular size were predictive of finding motile sperm. For patients with a prior history of PESA, repeat PESA has been reported on the ipsilateral testis with lower rates of sperm retrieval (26.3%).[20] One important consideration with PESA is that up to 25% of patients are unsuccessful in retrieval of sperm on their first attempt.[18] Patients then require a subsequent TESA or TESE. The rate of complications in PESA has been reported at 3.4% and includes pain, hydrocele, infection, and swelling.[21]

Testicular Sperm Aspiration

Retrieval of testicular sperm by percutaneous needle aspiration can be done in the outpatient setting with reliable results. TESA is most commonly performed on the day of egg retrieval because the amount of testicular tissue is minimal and may not be adequate for cryopreservation. However, Garg and colleagues[22] reported TESA outcomes in a retrospective case series of 40 patients from 2003 to 2007 and had adequate sperm retrieved for cryopreservation in 39 of 40 patients (97.5%) with no complications reported. In the modern-day evaluation of OA, TESA has continued utility as a diagnostic procedure. Among men with indeterminate clinical findings for OA versus NOA, it can be used to determine the presence or absence of spermatogenesis. There is also a role for TESA in the setting of a failed PESA. Often now termed a rescue TESA, this approach has been shown to have higher rates of successful sperm retrieval than PESA and represents an alternative backup option when PESA is unsuccessful. The quantity and motility of sperm in these cases tends to be lower than in a successful PESA.[7] Although TESA with proper technique results in rates of sperm recovery sufficient for ICSI in nearly 100% of men with azoospermia, other methods of sperm aspiration may produce superior samples with quantity more sufficient for cryopreservation.[23]

Percutaneous Vasal Sperm Aspiration

Vasal sperm aspiration is an option for men with obstruction at the level of the prostate or distal vas deferens, as well as in men with ejaculatory dysfunction. Reports of PVSA to achieve pregnancy have shown the technique to be highly successful. Qiu and colleagues[24] published their series of 26 patients with anejaculation who underwent sperm retrieval with PVSA followed by IUI. There was a 100% retrieval rate, with a pregnancy rate of 73.1%. Sperm was retrieved in sufficient volume and quality for IUI. Vasal sperm have the benefit of full maturation, making them an excellent sample for subsequent ICSI, IVF, IUI, or cryopreservation.[25] The site of obstruction is an important factor when PVSA is being considered, because healthy sperm in the scrotal vas are only likely to be present in cases of more distal obstruction, such as inguinal or ejaculatory duct obstruction.

Open Surgical Approaches to Sperm Retrieval

Although more invasive than percutaneous approaches, open surgical sperm extraction techniques play an important role in the diagnosis and management of men with OA. Both TESE and MESA reliably produce large numbers of sperm in men with OA.

Testicular Sperm Extraction

In men with OA, there is no consensus with respect to the superiority of sperm retrieved from the epididymis or testis in terms of IVF/ICSI outcomes, assuming sperm are successfully retrieved and readily available for use by the embryologist. Despite promising results of early studies of epididymal sperm, systematic reviews and meta-analyses have failed to find sufficient evidence to recommend one sperm retrieval technique rather than another.[26–28] Over time, TESE has become the most well-known and ubiquitous sperm retrieval technique, in large part because of the familiarity of urologists with testicular biopsy.

In men with OA, TESE produces a near-100% sperm retrieval rate. TESE has an important diagnostic role in men with normal testicular volume, palpable vasa deferentia, and normal or near-normal serum follicle-stimulating hormone levels. In addition to providing a tissue diagnosis of OA for men with no sperm in their samples, TESE allows extraction of a sufficient volume of sperm for cryopreservation. Any other method of percutaneous or open sperm retrieval that fails to identify sperm may be converted to a TESE with relative ease, and the ability to maneuver the conversion to a TESE should be made feasible within the chosen operative setting.

Microsurgical Epididymal Sperm Aspiration

MESA offers several benefits as a method of sperm retrieval in men with OA. Retrieval rates in appropriately selected men approach 100%. The number of sperm retrieved far exceeds those required for a single ICSI/IVF cycle and the sperm can be cryopreserved in 98% to 100% of cases. On average, MESA yields 15×10^6 to 95×10^6 total sperm with 15% to 42% total motility.[29,30] Combined with ICSI, epididymal sperm obtained by MESA has a clinical pregnancy rate of 42% to 60%.[28,30,31] Unlike TESE and percutaneous retrieval methods, MESA requires the use of an operative microscope and additional microsurgical training, which may limit its use by practitioners who either do not have access to a microscope or are less familiar with microsurgical techniques.

Minimally Invasive Epididymal Sperm Aspiration

Although MESA has emerged as reliable sperm retrieval procedure for men with OA, advances in technical aspects of the procedure have been designed to reduce the morbidity and complexity of the procedure. The mini-MESA, first described in 1998, decreased the incision size on a traditional MESA in hopes of improving postoperative pain and recovery time.[6,8] However, this did not address one of the main factors limiting the clinical use of MESA: the need for an operative microscope. Coward and Mills[7] further simplified the mini-MESA by performing the procedure solely under loupe magnification without compromising sperm yields. This approach is called a MIESA and can be performed either under oral or monitored anesthesia care (MAC) sedation.[7]

A MIESA begins much in the same way as a mini-MESA with a 1-cm transverse upper hemiscrotal incision. The testicle is exposed and an eyelid retractor is positioned within the tunica vaginalis to maintain exposure (**Fig. 2**). The caput of the epididymis is then rotated into the window opening and a 3-0 traction suture is placed in the upper third of the epididymis (**Fig. 3**).

The head of the epididymis is then gripped with the surgeon's nondominant hand as the assistant prepares a 1.0-mL tuberculin syringe with a 24-gauge angiocatheter tip primed with 0.1 mL of sperm wash medium. Additional syringes are prepared in similar fashion to allow smooth transition from one syringe to another. A 15° double-beveled straight ophthalmic blade is then passed into the epididymis in a single motion (**Fig. 4**). As the blade is slowly withdrawn, the epididymis is compressed and the assistant aspirates the expressed epididymal fluid. A single drop of the aspirate is evaluated in real time by a certified laboratory andrologist to confirm the presence of motile

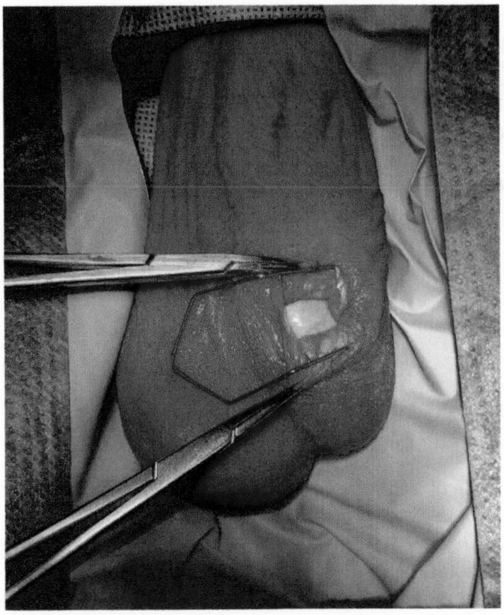

Fig. 2. Testis exposure using an eyelid retractor and mosquito forceps to facilitate closure.

sperm. If sperm are not immediately identified, progressive epididymotomies can be made proximally until high-quality motile sperm are extracted. Once high-quality sperm are identified, all proximal tubules are aspirated for cryopreservation.

FUTURE DIRECTIONS

The technical aspects of sperm retrieval have been honed throughout the years. Sperm samples sufficient for IVF or ICSI can now be reliably obtained from the epididymis or testicle via a variety of approaches, as described in this article. With continued success with sperm extraction and achievement of live birth via IVF/ICSI there has been an increasing focus on determining which sperm characteristics will lead to the best pregnancy and functional outcomes for offspring.

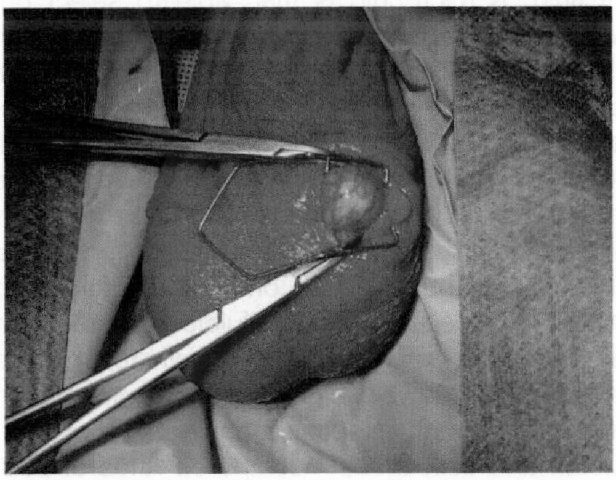

Fig. 3. Epididymal exposure.

Pregnancy outcomes between extraction sites have been examined in multiple studies with varied results. A meta-analysis of comparative studies in 2004 found there was no difference in IVF/ICSI outcomes between epididymal and testicular sperm.[32] A study in Denmark approached the questions of gamete source location from a developmental standpoint and compared functional outcomes of children born via IVF/ICSI using epididymal versus ejaculated sperm. Children born from epididymal sperm had equivalent motor skills, language skills, and rates of malformation compared with children born with ejaculated sperm.[32] This finding is in contrast with a 2012 *New England Journal of Medicine* article that found that children born via ICSI may be at higher risk for birth defects compared with children born naturally or even via conventional IVF.[33]

The theory behind the possibly increased risk of birth defects with ICSI is that, by performing ICSI, many of the intrinsic sperm selection processes are bypassed. In response to this concern, many of the emerging research studies and technologies are focused on sperm selection. Going beyond the traditional selection techniques used for ejaculated sperm, such as density-gradient centrifugation, sperm washing, and swim-up test, these emerging technologies include the role of DNA fragmentation as well as sperm selection with microfluidics and nanotechnology.

DNA Fragmentation

High rates of sperm DNA fragmentation are associated with worse outcomes in natural conception and IUI.[34] With respect to the impact of DNA fragmentation in IVF and ICSI, the data are more heterogeneous. Nevertheless, recent meta-analyses of the impact of high levels of DNA fragmentation on IVF outcomes have confirmed a negative effect. Zini[35] published a review of 11 studies and found a combined odds ratio (OR) of 1.70 (confidence interval [CI], 1.30–2.23) correlating high DNA fragmentation and failure to achieve pregnancy. An update to this review was published in 2017 with the addition of 9 additional articles. Again, higher levels of DNA fragmentation correlated with failure to achieve pregnancy (OR, 1.65; CI, 1.34–2.04).[36] The same meta-analysis also examined the effect of sperm DNA fragmentation on ICSI outcomes. Data combined from 24 studies found an OR of 1.31 (CI, 1.08–1.59) for ICSI failure among men with higher levels of DNA fragmentation.[36] Not all meta-analyses have confirmed the association of high DNA fragmentation and worse ICSI/IVF

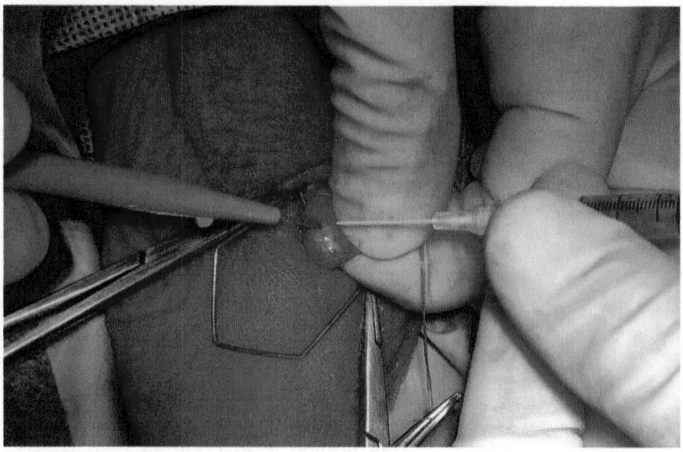

Fig. 4. Epididymotomy with ophthalmic blade followed by aspiration of epididymal fluid using 24-gauge angiocatheter on a syringe primed with sperm wash medium.

outcomes. Although Zhang and colleagues[37] found an association between DNA fragmentation greater than 27% and worse IVF outcomes, this did not hold true when studies were controlled for the type of fragmentation test used. More important than pregnancy rates as an outcome for IVF and ICSI are live-birth rates. Osman and colleagues[38] completed a systematic review and meta-analysis of live-birth rates with IVF or ICSI using sperm with high levels of DNA fragmentation. Greater fragmentation was associated with lower live-birth rates. Despite significant heterogeneity in individual studies, the predominant conclusion from meta-analyses and systematic reviews is that of an association between higher rates of sperm DNA fragmentation and poor outcomes with IVF and ICSI.[36]

Selection of testicular sperm may provide a means of reducing DNA fragmentation levels. In men with high levels of fragmentation in ejaculated samples, sperm retrieved directly from the testis has been shown to have lower levels of DNA fragmentation and better outcomes with ICSI.[21,39] Moskovtsev and colleagues[40] examined levels of DNA fragmentation in men with persistently high fragmentation following a 12-month course of oral antioxidants. Rates of DNA fragmentation were 3 times higher in ejaculated sperm compared with testicular sperm. A small series of men with OA found similar results. The study noted that DNA fragmentation rates were nearly twice as high in epididymal spermatozoa independent of the cause of OA.[41] There is some evidence of improved ICSI outcomes using testicular sperm in men with high levels of DNA fragmentation.[39] To date, only 1 prospective study has been published investigating treatment outcomes between ejaculated and testicular sperm. Esteves and colleagues[42] followed 172 men with high levels of DNA fragmentation undergoing ICSI. For the testicular sperm group, the relative risk for miscarriage was 0.29 (CI, 0.10–0.82) and the relative risk for live birth was 1.76 (CI, 1.15–2.70).

Emerging Techniques in Sperm Selection

Within a single sample, there is great heterogeneity with respect to the quality of individual sperm.[43] Since the introduction of ICSI in 1993, several techniques have been adopted to identify and select those sperm with the greatest fertilizing potential. These techniques range from conventional procedures such as sperm swim-up, glass wool filtration, and density-gradient centrifugation to more advanced techniques such as sperm magnetic sorting and high-magnification microscopy.[34,44] Microfluidics and nanotechnology are two emerging techniques with the potential to isolate good-quality sperm with a greater degree of precision.[45,46]

Microfluidics technology in sperm selection

The study of microfluidics involves the use of submillimeter channels to manipulate small volumes of fluid. A microchip is then able to select out various components of the fluid.[47] When run through a microfluidic device, healthy sperm is selected out into the chip from the channel. In general, there are 3 categories of microfluidic devices for sperm selection and sorting: those that isolate based on motility alone, those used for the observation and selection of individual sperm, and those that select sperm based on factors other than motility.[45] The use of microfluidic technology in sperm processing has been shown to produce samples with lower levels of DNA fragmentation and reactive oxygen species, and better motility.[48] Quinn and colleagues[49] compared rates of DNA fragmentation in sperm samples processed by microfluidic chip with those sorted through density-gradient centrifugation. Median DNA fragmentation index was 21% in the unprocessed semen sample, 6% in density-gradient centrifugation, and 0% by microfluidic chip. In a retrospective cohort study of couples undergoing IUI for infertility, microfluid sperm sorting resulted in higher ongoing pregnancy rates (15.03%) compared with density-gradient processed samples (9.09%). The OR of an ongoing pregnancy in the microfluidic group was 3.49 (CI, 1.12–10.89).[50] Further prospective, randomized trials are needed to assess the full extent and potential benefit of sperm selection with microfluidic technology.

Nanotechnology for sperm selection

Nanotechnology (the use of 1–100-nm materials with specific biological or chemical properties) has shown promise in sperm selection and labeling.[46] The field has expanded rapidly in biomedicine and now shows great potential in reproductive medicine.[51–53] Nanoparticles have the ability to remove less favorable sperm from a sample through a process termed nanopurification. For example, magnetic iron oxide nanoparticles have been shown to clear large semen volumes of acrosome-reacted or apoptotic spermatozoa.[46,54] This form of nanopurification has shown similar effects to established magnetic-assisted cell-sorting technologies.[46] Human studies examining the impact of nanopurification on fertility rates have not yet been completed. Nanotechnology has also been applied as a diagnostic tool for male infertility. Vidya and Saji[55] tethered heparin onto gold nanoparticles as a way to detect protamine levels in semen samples. As the most abundant nuclear protein in human sperm, protamine levels play an important role in the morphology of sperm,[56] which allows it to be used as a targeted biomarker to evaluate the fertility potential of a given semen sample. The binding of protamine to the heparin-tethered nanoparticles induces a color change to the naked eye that could be easily interpreted.[55] Although nanotechnology shows great potential in reproductive medicine, the human application of many of the nanoparticles in development has yet to be assessed.

SUMMARY

Men with OA have the benefit of a wide array of sperm extraction techniques that cater to the cause of their obstruction and produce reliable results in the hands of male fertility specialists. Percutaneous sperm aspiration techniques have remained highly effective tools with minimal modifications since their introduction. Open approaches to sperm extraction continue to shift toward less invasive practices in the hopes of facilitating their use in the clinic setting while minimizing patient morbidity. Innovations in sperm selection and purification may offer a means of improving the fertility potential of surgically retrieved specimens and address important emerging sperm parameters, including DNA fragmentation.

DISCLOSURE

The authors have nothing to disclose.

REFERENCES

1. Jarow JP, Espeland MA, Lipshultz LI. Evaluation of the azoospermic patient. J Urol 1989;142(1):62–5.
2. Wosnitzer MS, Goldstein M. Obstructive azoospermia. Urol Clin North Am 2014. https://doi.org/10.1016/j.ucl.2013.08.013.
3. Temple-Smith PD, Southwick GJ, Yates CA, et al. Human pregnancy by in vitro fertilization (IVF) using sperm aspirated from the epididymis. J In Vitro Fert Embryo Transf 1985. https://doi.org/10.1007/BF01131497.
4. Silber SJ, Balmaceda J, Borrero C, et al. Pregnancy with sperm aspiration from the proximal head of the epididymis: A new treatment for congenital absence of the vas deferens. Fertil Steril 1988. https://doi.org/10.1016/S0015-0282(16)60147-4.
5. Silber SJ, Nagy Z, Liu J, et al. The use of epididymal and testicular spermatozoa for intracytoplasmic sperm injection: the genetic implications for male infertility. Hum Reprod 1995;10(8):2031–43.
6. Nudell DM, Conaghan J, Pedersen RA, et al. The mini-micro-epididymal sperm aspiration for sperm retrieval: A study of urological outcomes. Hum Reprod 1998. https://doi.org/10.1093/humrep/13.5.1260.
7. Coward RM, Mills JN. A step-by-step guide to office-based sperm retrieval for obstructive azoospermia. Transl Androl Urol 2017. https://doi.org/10.21037/tau.2017.07.15.
8. Karpman E, Williams D. Techniques of sperm retrieval. In: Lipshultz LI, Howard SS, Niederberger CS, editors. Infertility in the male. 4th edition. New York: Cambridge University Press; 2009. p. 407–20.
9. Craft I, Shrivastav P, Quinton R, et al. Treatment of male infertility. Lancet 1994;344(8916):191–2.
10. Niederberger C, Pellicer A, Cohen J, et al. Forty years of IVF. Fertil Steril 2018;110(2):185–324.e5.
11. Schoysman R, Vanderzwalmen P, Nijs M, et al. Pregnancy after fertilisation with human testicular spermatozoa. Lancet 1993;342(8881):1237.

12. Foresta C, Varotto A, Scandellari C. Assessment of testicular cytology by fine needle aspiration as a diagnostic parameter in the evaluation of the azoospermic subject. Fertil Steril 1992;57(4):858–65.
13. Bourne H, Watkins W, Speirs A, et al. Pregnancies after intracytoplasmic injection of sperm collected by fine needle biopsy of the testis. Fertil Steril 1995;64(2):433–6.
14. Jensen CFS, Ohl DA, Hiner MR, et al. Multiple needle-pass percutaneous testicular sperm aspiration as first-line treatment in azoospermic men. Andrology 2016;4(2):257–62.
15. Lewin A, Weiss DB, Friedler S, et al. Delivery following intracytoplasmic injection of mature sperm cells recovered by testicular fine needle aspiration in a case of hypergonadotropic azoospermia due to maturation arrest. Hum Reprod 1996;11(4):769–71.
16. Schlegel PN. Testicular sperm extraction: microdissection improves sperm yield with minimal tissue excision. Hum Reprod 1999;14(1):131–5.
17. Qiu Y, Su Q, Wang S, et al. Percutaneous vasal sperm aspiration and intrauterine insemination in the treatment of obstructive azoospermia. Fertil Steril 1997;68(6):1135–8.
18. Yafi FA, Zini A. Percutaneous epididymal sperm aspiration for men with obstructive azoospermia: predictors of successful sperm retrieval. Urology 2013;82:341–4.
19. Collins GN, Critchlow JD, Lau MW, et al. Open versus closed epididymal sperm retrieval in men with secondarily obstructed vasal systems–a preliminary report. Br J Urol 1996;78(3):437–9.
20. Pasqualotto FF, Rossi-Ferragut LM, Rocha CC, et al. The efficacy of repeat percutaneous epididymal sperm aspiration procedures. J Urol 2003. https://doi.org/10.1097/01.ju.0000066849.32466.2b.
21. Esteves SC, Lee W, Benjamin DJ, et al. Reproductive potential of men with obstructive azoospermia undergoing percutaneous sperm retrieval and intracytoplasmic sperm injection according to the cause of obstruction. J Urol 2013. https://doi.org/10.1016/j.juro.2012.08.084.
22. Garg T, LaRosa C, Strawn E, et al. Outcomes After Testicular Aspiration and Testicular Tissue Cryopreservation for Obstructive Azoospermia and Ejaculatory Dysfunction. J Urol 2008;180(6):2577–80.
23. Tournaye H, Clasen K, Aytoz A, et al. Fine needle aspiration versus open biopsy for testicular sperm recovery: A controlled study in azoospermic patients with normal spermatogenesis. Hum Reprod 1998; 13(4):901–4.
24. Qiu Y, Wang SM, Yang DT, et al. Percutaneous vasal sperm aspiration and intrauterine insemination for infertile males with anejaculation. Fertil Steril 2003; 79(3):618–20.
25. Bachtell NE, Conaghan J, Turek PJ. The relative viability of human spermatozoa from the vas deferens, epididymis and testis before and after cryopreservation. Hum Reprod 1999;14(12): 3048–51.
26. Palermo GD, Schlegel PN, Hariprashad JJ, et al. Fertilization and pregnancy outcome with intracytoplasmic sperm injection for azoospermic men. Hum Reprod 1999;14:741–8. Available at: https://academic.oup.com/humrep/article-abstract/14/3/741/632914.
27. Van Peperstraten A, Proctor M, Johnson N, et al. Techniques for surgical retrieval of sperm prior to ICSI for azoospermia. Cochrane Database Syst Rev 2008;(2):CD002807.
28. Nicopoullos JDM, Gilling-Smith C, Almeida PA, et al. Use of surgical sperm retrieval in azoospermic men: A meta-analysis. Fertil Steril 2004. https://doi.org/10.1016/j.fertnstert.2004.02.116.
29. Bernie AM, Ramasamy R, Stember DS, et al. Microsurgical epididymal sperm aspiration: Indications, techniques and outcomes. Asian J Androl 2013. https://doi.org/10.1038/aja.2012.114.
30. Hibi H, Sumitomo M, Fukunaga N, et al. Superior clinical pregnancy rates after microsurgical epididymal sperm aspiration. Reprod Med Biol 2018. https://doi.org/10.1002/rmb2.12069.
31. Bromage SJ, Falconer DA, Lieberman BA, et al. Sperm retrieval rates in subgroups of primary azoospermic males. Eur Urol 2007;51(2):534–9 [discussion: 539–40].
32. Woldringh GH, Horvers M, Janssen AJWM, et al. Follow-up of children born after ICSI with epididymal spermatozoa. Hum Reprod 2011;26(7): 1759–67.
33. Davies MJ, Moore VM, Willson KJ, et al. Reproductive technologies and the risk of birth defects. N Engl J Med 2012;366(19):1803–13.
34. Agarwal A, Cho C-L, Esteves SC. Should we evaluate and treat sperm DNA fragmentation? Curr Opin Obstet Gynecol 2016;28(3):164–71.
35. Zini A. Are sperm chromatin and DNA defects relevant in the clinic? Syst Biol Reprod Med 2011;57: 78–85.
36. Simon L, Zini A, Dyachenko A, et al. A systematic review and meta-analysis to determine the effect of sperm DNA damage on in vitro fertilization and intracytoplasmic sperm injection outcome. Asian J Androl 2017;19(1):80–90.
37. Zhang Z, Zhu L, Jiang H, et al. Sperm DNA fragmentation index and pregnancy outcome after IVF or ICSI: a meta-analysis. J Assist Reprod Genet 2015;32(1):17–26.
38. Osman A, Alsomait H, Seshadri S, et al. The effect of sperm DNA fragmentation on live birth rate after IVF or ICSI: a systematic review and meta-analysis. Reprod Biomed Online 2015;30(2):120–7.
39. Esteves SC, Roque M, Garrido N. Use of testicular sperm for intracytoplasmic sperm injection in men

with high sperm DNA fragmentation: a SWOT analysis. Asian J Androl 2018;20(1):1–8.
40. Moskovtsev SI, Jarvi K, Mullen JBM, et al. Testicular spermatozoa have statistically significantly lower DNA damage compared with ejaculated spermatozoa in patients with unsuccessful oral antioxidant treatment. Fertil Steril 2010;93(4):1142–6.
41. Hammoud I, Bailly M, Bergere M, et al. Testicular Spermatozoa Are of Better Quality Than Epididymal Spermatozoa in Patients With Obstructive Azoospermia. Urology 2017. https://doi.org/10.1016/j.urology.2016.11.019.
42. Esteves SC, Sánchez-Martín F, Sánchez-Martín P, et al. Comparison of reproductive outcome in oligozoospermic men with high sperm DNA fragmentation undergoing intracytoplasmic sperm injection with ejaculated and testicular sperm. Fertil Steril 2015;104(6):1398–405.
43. Jeyendran RS, Schrader SM, Van Der Ven HH, et al. Association of the in-vitro fertilizing capacity of human spermatozoa with sperm morphology as assessed by three classification systems. Hum Reprod 1986;1(5):305–8.
44. Jeyendran RS, Caroppo E, Rouen A, et al. Selecting the most competent sperm for assisted reproductive technologies. Fertil Steril 2019;111(5):851–63.
45. Samuel R, Feng H, Jafek A, et al. Microfluidic-based sperm sorting & analysis for treatment of male infertility. Transl Androl Urol 2018;7:S336–47.
46. Feugang JM. Novel agents for sperm purification, sorting, and imaging. Mol Reprod Dev 2017;84(9): 832–41.
47. Whitesides GM. The origins and the future of microfluidics. Nature 2006;442(7101):368–73.
48. Asghar W, Velasco V, Kingsley JL, et al. Selection of Functional Human Sperm with Higher DNA Integrity and Fewer Reactive Oxygen Species. Adv Healthc Mater 2014;3(10):1671–9.
49. Quinn MM, Jalalian L, Ribeiro S, et al. Microfluidic sorting selects sperm for clinical use with reduced DNA damage compared to density gradient centrifugation with swim-up in split semen samples. Hum Reprod 2018;33(8):1388–93.
50. Gode F, Bodur T, Gunturkun F, et al. Comparison of microfluid sperm sorting chip and density gradient methods for use in intrauterine insemination cycles. Fertil Steril 2019. https://doi.org/10.1016/j.fertnstert.2019.06.037.
51. Barkalina N, Jones C, Coward K. Nanomedicine and mammalian sperm: Lessons from the porcine model. Theriogenology 2016;85(1):74–82.
52. Feugang JM, Youngblood RC, Greene JM, et al. Self-illuminating quantum dots for non-invasive bioluminescence imaging of mammalian gametes. J Nanobiotechnology 2015;13(1). https://doi.org/10.1186/s12951-015-0097-1.
53. Sutovsky P, Kennedy CE. Biomarker-based nanotechnology for the improvement of reproductive performance in beef and dairy cattle. Ind Biotechnol 2013;9(1):24–30.
54. Durfey CL, Swistek SE, Liao SF, et al. Nanotechnology-based approach for safer enrichment of semen with best spermatozoa. J Anim Sci Biotechnol 2019;10(1). https://doi.org/10.1186/s40104-018-0307-4.
55. Vidya R, Saji A. Naked eye detection of infertility based on sperm protamine-induced aggregation of heparin gold nanoparticles. Anal Bioanal Chem 2018;410(13):3053–8.
56. Oliva R, Dixon GH. Vertebrate protamine genes and the histone-to-protamine replacement reaction. Prog Nucleic Acid Res Mol Biol 1991;40:25–94.

Testicular Mapping
A Roadmap to Sperm Retrieval in Nonobstructive Azoospermia?

Akash A. Kapadia, MD*, Thomas J. Walsh, MD, MS

KEYWORDS

• Testicular mapping • MicroTESE • Azoospermia • FNA mapping • Testis biopsy • Sperm retrieval

KEY POINTS

- Men with nonobstructive azoospermia (NOA) should undergo complete genetic testing before discussion of surgical sperm retrieval.
- Offered treatment pathways may involve testicular mapping followed by sperm retrieval or upfront sperm retrieval and should include discussion of both advantages and disadvantages.
- The couple should be encouraged to help guide the decision.

SETTING THE STAGE

The diagnosis of azoospermia must be confirmed with 2 separate semen analyses demonstrating complete absence of sperm using high-powered microscopy. Once the diagnosis of nonobstructive azoospermia (NOA) has been confirmed with thorough history, physical examination, and hormonal testing, important considerations must then be made in order to guide a couple through their journey to parenthood. The couple should be made aware that assisted reproduction, whether through partner or donor sperm, traditional adoption, and embryo adoption, is the pathway forward. Foremost, genetic testing in the form of karyotype and Y-chromosome microdeletion (YCMD) should be obtained for the purposes of counseling and prognostication. Both Klinefelter syndrome (KS) and YCMD have a prevalence of approximately 10% in men with NOA.[1–3] Guiding the couple on the probability of finding sperm may start with a discussion of genetic evaluation in patients who accept this testing. In patients without an identifiable cause of NOA, the natural follow-up questions are: *what are my chances of finding sperm?* and *what is the best approach to finding sperm?*

Several studies have investigated noninvasive predictors of sperm retrieval. Colpi and colleagues[4] and Ghalayini and colleagues[5] have shown that increased follicle stimulating hormone (FSH) levels are associated with decreased retrieval success regardless of the type of retrieval procedure. In the same studies, Colpi could not show a significant relation between testicular volume and sperm retrieval; however, Ghalayini demonstrated a positive correlation between testicular volume and retrieval success. On the contrary, Ramasamy and colleagues[6] in their large cohort did not show a correlation between high FSH levels and sperm-retrieval failure via microdissection testicular sperm extraction (microTESE). A composite analysis of sperm-retrieval data suggests that testicular volume and hormonal values alone do not exhibit reliable predictive value in retrieval success.

Testicular histology is the most reliable predictor of sperm-retrieval success. Men with the least severe form of spermatogenic dysfunction (ie, hypospermatogenesis) demonstrate a retrieval rate of 80% to 98%, whereas those with the most severe form of spermatogenic dysfunction (ie, sertoli cell only syndrome [SCOS] or germ

Department of Urology, University of Washington, 1959 Northeast Pacific Street, Box 356510, Seattle, WA 98195, USA
* Corresponding author.
E-mail address: kapadiaa@uw.edu

Urol Clin N Am 47 (2020) 157–164
https://doi.org/10.1016/j.ucl.2019.12.013

cell aplasia) have a success rate of 5% to 24%. Most notably, those with less severe forms of spermatogenic dysfunction demonstrate a high retrieval rate even with the least invasive techniques of sperm retrieval.[7–9] There are several limitations of testicular histology, however. First, the performance of biopsy introduces the risk associated with a diagnostic procedure. As it is known, an open biopsy may then lead to a second invasive procedure for sperm retrieval. Second, and perhaps even more important, there is evidence of high discordance in histologic diagnosis among pathologists. In 2003, Cooperberg and colleagues[10] reported significant intraobserver variability between initial histologic diagnosis and subsequent review diagnosis from 1 institution to another that resulted in clinically significant changes to management of 27% of patients. Last, it is well established that spermatogenesis can be focal and sporadic, and therefore, limited sampling via a single or multiple "random" biopsies may still lead to incomplete information on spermatogenesis while introducing additional risk to patients.[11]

Sousa and colleagues[8] reported significant histologic variability in patients with previously diagnosed "sertoli cell only syndrome," because nearly 40% of the men had a combination of maturation arrest, early, or late spermiogenesis in the study cohort. As a result, sperm retrieval in their patients ranged from 5% to 98% via conventional testicular sperm extraction (cTESE). Thus, it has been suggested that focal spermatogenesis in patients with histologically diagnosed "SCOS" cannot be reliably predicted even in the setting of multiple random biopsies. Ramasamy and Schlegel[12] have described sperm-retrieval rates (SRR) as high as 51% with microTESE in patients with prior biopsies, albeit demonstrating lower retrieval rates and poorer outcomes in cases with increasing negative prior biopsies. Furthermore, the same group reported a retrieval rate of 37% in patients with "SCOS" and at least 1 prior negative biopsy. Therefore, when evaluating predictive factors for sperm retrieval, it is apparent that although histology can guide sperm retrieval in many patients with less severe forms of spermatogenic failure, it does not reliably predict absence of spermatogenesis in those with "SCOS" diagnosed from a traditional, focal or multifocal, biopsy.

A provider may then ask: *How do I guide my patients with NOA toward their treatment goals?* Because of the historically poor predictive tools for successful sperm retrieval, 2 care pathways have emerged: *Upfront testicular sperm retrieval versus testicular mapping guided sperm retrieval.*

UPFRONT TESTICULAR SPERM RETRIEVAL

There are 2 accepted forms of sperm-retrieval techniques: percutaneous and open.

Percutaneous Retrieval

During a percutaneous procedure for NOA, sperm is aspirated with a moderately large-gauge needle or angiocatheter that is inserted percutaneously after an adequate spermatic cord block. It may also be performed with adjunctive sedation. Using a standard Luer-Lock or Cameco piston syringe to generate suction, the needle is oscillated in the same plane to release a substantial conglomerate of testicular tubules. These tubules are released at the skin and transferred into buffer media for morcellation, analysis, and storage.[13] Patients with NOA are generally reported to have lower success rates with upfront percutaneous techniques (11%–47%) compared with open techniques (16%–63%).[14–17] Mercan and colleagues[15] reported an SRR of 14% with percutaneous aspiration in their cohort of 452 men with NOA. Those who had a failed aspiration (testicular sperm aspiration [TESA]) went on to have a cTESE in the same setting with an overall SRR of 64.4%. Men with a successful aspiration in their cohort had a much higher likelihood of hypospermatogenesis as the predominant histopathology and were much less likely to have maturation arrest or germ cell aplasia. Vicari and colleagues[14] described a much higher rate of SRR with aspiration at 47.3%, albeit with a smaller cohort of NOA. Similar to the prior study, their results showed that aspiration was successful in 100% of men who had diagnostic biopsies demonstrating hypospermatogenesis or maturation arrest with focal spermatogenesis, but the success rates with this technique were lower in complete maturation arrest (42.3%), SCOS (14.3%), and SCOS with focal spermatogenesis (0%).

Table 1 outlines outcomes observed through percutaneous procedures.

Open Retrieval

Open testicular sperm extraction (TESE) can be accomplished using 2 main methods: conventional TESE (via single or multiple random/directed biopsies) and microTESE.

Conventional testicular sperm extraction

cTESE is distinct from a percutaneous procedure in that it involves incision of the tunica albuginea in order to obtain tissue. It is distinct from microTESE in that it does not involve the use of high-powered microscopy and testicular bivalving (see later discussion) in order to guide retrieval. As a result, testicular tissue is retrieved via a single

Table 1
Sperm-retrieval outcomes from percutaneous procedures (testicular sperm aspiration)

Author, Year	Case (n)	SRR (%)
Friedler et al,[17] 1997	37	11
Ezeh et al,[16] 1998	35	14
Mercan et al,[15] 2000	452	14
Vicari et al,[14] 2001	55	47.3

Data from Refs. [14–16]

incision or multiple incisions based on surgeon preference. Tubular characteristics are not factored in tissue retrieval, as is the case with microTESE. SRRs from various studies are outlined in **Table 2**. In a 2006 study, Vernaeve and colleagues[18] reported an overall SRR of 49% with 41% success on first attempt. This study showed high SRR in those men who underwent repeat cTESE with a second attempt resulting in 75% SRR (n = 77), third attempt resulting in 82% SRR (n = 28), and fourth attempt resulting in 100% SRR (n = 11). On pathology review, they found a 98.9% SRR in men with hypospermatogenesis, of which all 57 men undergoing their first cTESE had successful retrieval. On the contrary, in men with "SCOS," the SSR was 38.7% on first attempt and 77.6% on second attempt.[18] As before, SCOS is placed in quotes, because clearly, if sperm are retrieved, this is not the true diagnosis. From this study, and across all studies with available pathology, it is once again clear that men with hypospermatogenesis have reliably and reproducibly high SRRs using conventional methods of retrieval. However, the efficacy of these methods decreases substantially in cases of severe spermatogenic dysfunction.

Microdissection testicular sperm extraction

First described in 1999 by Schlegel,[19] microTESE has suggested promising results in men with NOA when compared with cTESE. In most scenarios, microTESE is performed under general anesthesia. The testes are examined one at a time, with most surgeons preferring to initiate exploration in the larger of the two. After delivery of the testis, the tunica albuginea is incised equatorially toward the mediastinum testis bilaterally, thereby avoiding the traverse of areas rich in vascularity. Upon completing the "bivalving" of the testis, high-powered microscopy enables the systematic examination of the seminiferous tubules in each of the testicular lobules. Dilated opaque tubules are sought in a sea of collapsed or obliterated tubular architecture. Once promising tubules are harvested, they are placed in a buffer,

Table 2
Sperm-retrieval outcomes from conventional testicular sperm extraction

Author, Year	Case (n)	SRR (%)
Schlegel,[19] 1999	22	45
Amer et al,[20] 2000	100	30
Mercan et al,[15] 2000	389	59
Okada et al,[21] 2002	24	16.7
Tsujimura et al,[22] 2002	37	35.1
Ramasamy et al,[23] 2005	83	32
Vernaeve et al,[18] 2006	628	49
Ghalayini et al,[5] 2011	68	38.2

Data from Refs. [5,15,18–23]

morcellated, and examined by an andrologist or embryologist in real time for the presence of sperm. A decision regarding exploration of the contralateral testis is made based on quantity and quality of obtained sperm. Hemostasis is attained with bipolar electrocautery; the tunica albuginea is securely closed, and the testis is returned to the tunica vaginalis (**Fig. 1**).[24]

Several studies over the last 2 decades have shown higher rates of sperm retrieval using microTESE (**Table 3**), and these results have been confirmed in a recent metaanalysis.[25] Another metaanalysis that appraised all 3 techniques (TESA, cTESE, and microTESE) reported that microTESE was 1.5 times more likely to result in successful retrieval compared with cTESE, and in turn, cTESE is 2 times more likely to result in successful retrieval compared with TESA.[26] All indications suggest that microTESE results in SRRs may be clinically significant for patients. When evaluating these data, however, one must also consider an inspection under the microscope. Three studies directly compared SRRs in patients with hypospermatogenesis undergoing cTESE and microTESE. Okada and colleagues[21] and Tsujimura and colleagues[22] did not demonstrate statistical significance in SRRs within their cohorts. Ramasamy and colleagues[23] did show a significant difference in favor of microTESE in their cohort (50% vs 81%). SRRs in hypospermatogenesis across all studies ranged from 81% to 100% with microTESE, and from 50% to 84% with cTESE. Four studies directly compared SRRs in patients previously diagnosed with "SCOS." In their cohorts, Okada and colleagues[21] and Ghalayini and colleagues5 demonstrated statistical and clinical superiority with microTESE. Overall, SRRs in "SCOS" ranged from 22.5% to 41% with microTESE, and from 6.3% to 29% with cTESE. Overall, the results give a sense that

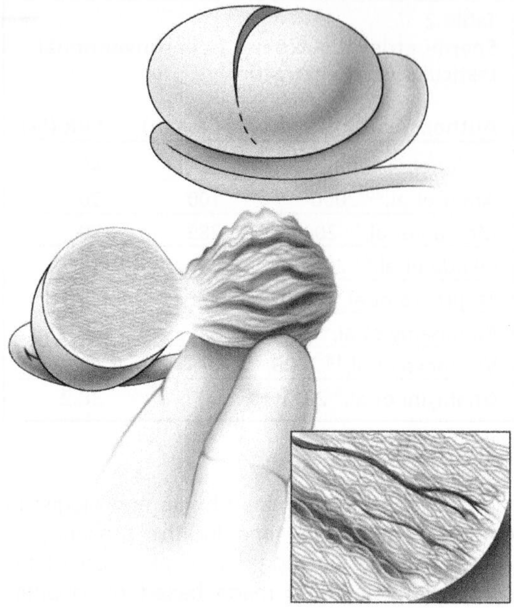

Fig. 1. The testicle is delivered through a scrotal incision. An equatorial incision is made in the tunica albuginea, thus bivalving the testis. The seminiferous tubules are then examined for dilated tubules under an operating microscope. These dilated tubules are more likely to contain sperm and should be harvested to be processed by the embryology/andrology team. The tunica albuginea is then closed with a running suture. The testicle is placed back in the scrotum and the tunica vaginalis, dartos, and skin layers are closed. (*From* Ramasamy R, Yagan N, Schlegel PN. Structural and functional changes to the testis after conventional versus microdissection testicular sperm extraction. Urology. 2005;65(5)1190–1194; with permission.)

men with severe pathologic condition would certainly benefit from a technologically advanced, skill-intensive procedure such as microTESE.

Complications of Sperm Retrieval

In addition to improved SRR, microTESE may result in less loss of tissue from the testis.

Table 3
Sperm-retrieval outcomes from microdissection testicular sperm extraction

Author, Year	Case (n)	SRR (%)
Schlegel,[19] 1999	27	63
Amer et al,[20] 2000	100	47
Tsujimura et al,[22] 2002	56	42.9
Okada et al,[21] 2002	74	44.6
Ramasamy et al,[23] 2005	460	57
Ishikawa et al,[27] 2010	150	42
Ghalayini et al,[5] 2011	65	56.9

Data from Refs. [5,19–23,27]

Studies have reported testicular mass reduction ranging from 150 to 720 mg with cTESE. In comparison, mass reduction of approximately 10 to 300 mg has been reported in microTESE.[18,19,28] Harrington and colleagues[29] reported a 29% rate of intratesticular hematoma in cTESE, which may lead to high rates of scarring and additional volume loss. Since then, studies have evaluated patients with serial ultrasound studies to quantify volume loss. In a prospective study of 60 patients, Amer and colleagues[20] described a higher rate of persistent echogenic foci in patients who underwent cTESE compared with microTESE; however, there were no cases of permanent testicular devascularization, as has been previously reported by Schlegel and Su.[28] Subsequently, in a study of 147 men, Okada and colleagues[21] reported higher rates of persistent findings of hematoma, chronic changes, and lower testicular volumes at 6 months with cTESE compared with microTESE, although a decrease in testosterone and need for testosterone replacement were not different between the comparison groups. Ramasamy and colleagues[23] evaluated 435 men with NOA and also found a higher rate of focal hypoechoic changes on ultrasound at 6 months with cTESE. The study also revealed a 20% decline in serum testosterone from baseline at 6 months in both groups with just more than one-third of men returning to 95% of preoperative testosterone levels at 18 months.

Similarly, others have evaluated the risk of hypogonadism following sperm-retrieval procedures. Most of the studies find a higher rate of androgen decline in patients with KS who typically start at a lower total testosterone, and return to 50% to 75% of preoperative values.[30] These patients should be monitored closely for symptoms of hypogonadism. In NOA patients without KS, studies show initial significant decline followed by normalization of total testosterone at 12 to 18 months.[21–23,31,32] Although there are measurable ultrasound and hormonal changes in both the short and the long term, it remains to be seen whether these findings correlate with clinical outcomes of hypogonadism.

It is evident that even with the most advanced form of sperm-retrieval techniques, nearly 40% to 50% of men with NOA may undergo an invasive procedure only to return empty-handed. A male infertility specialist must wonder how these men can be identified in order to avoid unnecessary surgery in both the male and in many cases the female partner. By the same principle, can success be maximized with sperm retrieval while minimizing harm to the patient?

TESTICULAR MAPPING

The questions raised above are the guiding principles that led to the conception and development of testicular mapping. In 1997, Turek was the first US urologist to describe testicular fine needle aspiration (FNA) mapping as a way to improve diagnostic accuracy compared with testicular biopsy/histology based on the knowledge that spermatogenesis is focal and sporadic.[11] Testicular FNA mapping is performed with a spermatic cord block using a 23- or 24-gauge needle on a 10-mL syringe and a suctioning syringe holder (Cameco). Aspiration sites are planned depending on the testis size, but typically range between 12 and 18 sites. Given the small needle gauge, only a miniscule number of tubules are extracted and deposited on microscope slides. The seminiferous tubules are smeared onto the microscope slide using standard cytologic principles and fixed with either 95% ethyl alcohol or other suitable fixative. Aspirated seminiferous tubules undergo staining and are examined by a cytopathologist or laboratory andrologist for the presence of sperm. Specimen handling, processing, and interpretation require expertise in cytologic techniques. Patient recovery is rapid, and postprocedural pain is managed with no-narcotic pain medications (**Fig. 2**).[33]

In their 1997 pilot study, Turek and colleagues[11] described 16 patients who underwent matched open testicular biopsies and FNA mapping. Testis mapping was more sensitive than open biopsy and equally specific in detecting sperm. Numerous studies have now shown a very high concordance rate between FNA cytology and open biopsy histology, allowing for high reliability in prognostication of patients.[33–36] In a subsequent study, Turek and colleagues[33] reported the identification of sperm via FNA in 27.1% of men who had a negative previous biopsy.[37] This finding is further strengthened by findings showing sperm detection rates of 47% in men who underwent FNA at 7 sites per testicle, increasing to 52% with 14 sites per testicle, findings that are similar to rates of sperm retrieval when microTESE is performed.[38]

Of the men who had detectable sperm, FNA-directed TESE were performed under local anesthesia with a mean 3.1 biopsies per patient and 72 mg of tissue removed. Sufficient sperm was obtained for all oocytes in 95% of in vitro fertilization (IVF) cycles (20/21).[39] Using an alternative aspiration technique, Lewin and colleagues[40] demonstrated a 58.8% sperm detection rate with FNA when averaging 15 sites per testicle, indicating that increasing number of sampling per testicle correlates with higher sperm detection rate. Once again, these studies seem to confirm a success rate of sperm identification and subsequent retrieval that may be comparable to that of upfront microTESE.

Importantly, the information obtained via the FNA map may help to tailor sperm retrieval that yields the greatest success while minimizing invasiveness for the patient. In a series of 132 NOA cases with FNA mapping, 45 patients underwent directed TESA or TESE, whereas 14 underwent directed microTESE. Jad and Turek[41] found a retrieval rate of 98% (44/45 cases) in the TESA/TESE cohort, whereas microTESE resulted in 86% success (12/14 cases). In addition, all microdissection cases in this series of previously FNA mapped patients were unilateral and involved sperm retrieval from only 1 testicle. Overall, sufficient sperm was obtained in 95% of cases. As such, the testis map may offer a less invasive

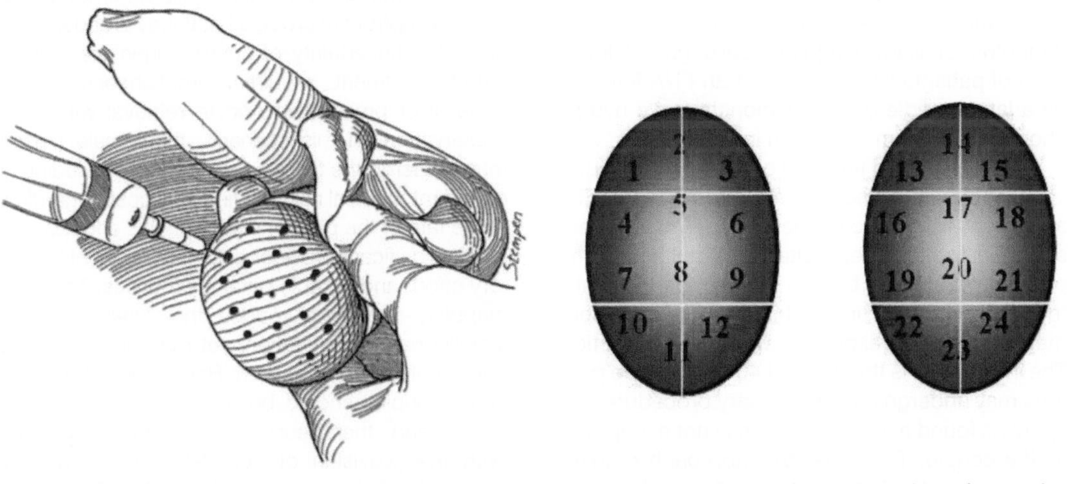

Fig. 2. FNA mapping procedure and mapping template. *From* Beliveau ME, Turek PJ. The value of testicular "mapping" in men with non-obstructive azoospermia. Asian J Androl. 2011; 13(2): 225-230; with permission.

form of identifying areas of spermatogenesis, if present, and a guide for efficient, targeted, and less invasive future sperm-retrieval procedures.

An additional area of testicular mapping utilization is in cases of failed microTESE when a patient desires further investigation. In a recent study, Jarvis and colleagues[42] retrospectively identified 82 patients who had a failed microTESE and subsequently underwent FNA-guided testicular mapping. Of these, 24 (29%) men had at least 1 FNA site that was positive for sperm. Fifteen men then underwent a sperm-retrieval procedure with successful retrieval in all, as well as successful cryopreservation for future use in 10 (67%). Similar studies in patients who undergo repeat microTESE after a failed microTESE revealed success in 30% to 50% of patients. Talas and colleagues[43] described 3 of 5 patients who had a successful repeat microTESE following initial failure, whereas Morris and colleagues[44] reported 3 of 9 patients who had successful repeat microTESE. Clearly, these findings speak to the potential variation with how microTESE is performed. In this setting, testicular mapping may help select patients who could then go on to have a directed microTESE at a higher success rate, while avoiding a second invasive procedure in those with unfavorable findings.

Testicular mapping has been reported to be well tolerated and with a minimal complication profile. Lewin and colleagues[40] demonstrated a 7% rate of intratesticular bleeding on ultrasound 30 minutes following the procedure, which did not result in clinically measurable changes in postprocedural care. In extrapolating outcomes after large needle aspirations, Westlander and colleagues[45] found no changes in FSH or testosterone levels 3 months following the procedure. These investigators found no change in testicular volumes; however, 4 patients (6%) had focal echogenic intratesticular lesions with 3 of 4 seeing resolution in 6 to 9 months. Similarly, Carpi and colleagues[46] found 11% of patients who underwent an FNA followed by a large-needle biopsy demonstrated a hypoechoic area of 1 cm or less on imaging.

The physical and financial burden on the couple is also of importance. The upfront microTESE approach, as classically described, implies fresh sperm utilization, necessitating simultaneous or prior egg retrieval by the female partner, and thereby resulting in distribution of precious manpower and resources within the practice. The implication is that at least 40% of female partners may undergo an unnecessary procedure if no sperm is found and donor sperm is not acceptable to the couple. Therefore, this approach requires extensive upfront counseling of couples, and detailed discussion of the "what if" scenarios. Finally, from a cost-effectiveness standpoint, preliminary cost analysis models looking at incremental cost-effectiveness ratio have shown that testicular mapping may yield a slightly lower SRR, but is more cost-effective than microTESE.[47]

In summary, FNA-guided testicular mapping may help to avoid several pitfalls encountered with random biopsies. It relies on cytology for sperm detection, hence avoiding problems with histologic variability and markedly increasing sensitivity. Furthermore, it demonstrates concordance to histologic findings, lending credibility to cytologic findings. Importantly, using a grid technique (as described in later discussion) provides direct knowledge of present or absent mature spermatozoa (as well as immature sperm forms) at any given site. In a scenario whereby a patient demonstrates diffuse hypospermatogenesis on the testis map, it arms the provider with options of performing less invasive and less costly retrieval procedures, like TESA or cTESE. On the contrary, when faced with complete absence of spermatogenesis, it allows a provider the confidence and assurance of appropriate patient counseling.

Patient-Centered Approach to Care

Many in andrology will agree that providing the best care means coming to learn about goals and values of the couples for whom they are caring. Various cultural, psychosocial, emotional, financial, and personal factors may become apparent during a patient visit, which may guide the shared decision-making process. Patients should be apprised of not just success and complication rates of the care pathways but also the emotional and economic burdens of what is to come. Men often endure the easier burden of the two, and this should be emphasized. When an upfront microTESE pathway is undertaken, given the uncertainty of spermatogenesis, coordinated treatment requires simultaneous oocyte retrieval or preemptive oocyte retrieval with cryopreservation. In this scenario, the female partner must undergo the full process with IVF, including its attendant medical risk and financial cost, regardless of the fate of the partner's sperm. This endeavor requires significant provider planning, hours of laboratory effort, and notable patient expenses. Testicular mapping may help reduce the "unknown" and simplify care coordination, yet may place a higher burden of care on the man. Regardless of the scenario, couples should be presented with all diagnostic and therapeutic sperm-retrieval options. With the provision of complete information, the couple should be empowered to make informed decisions regarding their care.

DISCLOSURE

The authors of this article have no financial conflict of interest.

REFERENCES

1. Barr ML. The natural history of Klinefelter's syndrome. Fertil Steril 1966;17:429–41.
2. Visootsak J, Graham JM Jr. Klinefelter syndrome and other sex chromosomal aneuploidies. Orphanet J Rare Dis 2006;24:1–42.
3. Stahl PJ, Mielnik A, Schlegel PN, et al. A decade of experience emphasizes that testing for Y chromosome microdeletions (YCM) is essential in men with azoospermia and severe oligospermia. Fertil Steril 2008;90:S319.
4. Colpi GM, Colpi EM, Piediferro G, et al. Microsurgical TESE versus conventional TESE for ICSI in non-obstructive azoospermia: a randomized controlled study. Reprod Biomed Online 2009;18:315–9.
5. Ghalayini IF, Al-Ghazo MA, Hani OB, et al. Clinical comparison of conventional testicular sperm extraction and microdissection techniques for non-obstructive azoospermia. J Clin Med Res 2011;3:123–31.
6. Ramasamy R, Lin K, Gosden LV, et al. High serum FSH levels in men with nonobstructive azoospermia does not affect success of microdissection testicular sperm extraction. Fertil Steril 2009;92:590–3.
7. Seo JT, Ko WJ. Predictive factors of successful testicular sperm recovery in non-obstructive azoospermia patients. Int J Androl 2001;24:306–10.
8. Sousa M, Cremades N, Silva J, et al. Predictive value of testicular histology in secretory azoospermic subgroups and clinical outcome after microinjection of fresh and frozen-thawed sperm and spermatids. Hum Reprod 2002;17:1800–10.
9. Su LM, Palermo GD, Goldstein M, et al. Testicular sperm extraction with intracytoplasmic sperm injection for nonobstructive azoospermia: testicular histology can predict success of sperm retrieval. J Urol 1999;161:112–6.
10. Cooperberg MR, Chi T, Jad A, et al. Variability in testis biopsy interpretation: implications for male infertility care in the era of intracytoplasmic sperm injection. Fertil Steril 2005;84:672–7.
11. Turek PJ, Cha I, Ljung B-M. Systematic fine-needle aspiration of the testis: correlation to biopsy and results of organ "mapping" for mature sperm in azoospermic men. Urology 1997;49:743–8.
12. Ramasamy R, Schlegel PN. Microdissection testicular sperm extraction: effect of prior biopsy on success of sperm retrieval. J Urol 2007;177:1447–9.
13. Gorgy A, Podsiadly BT, Bates S, et al. Testicular sperm aspiration (TESA): the appropriate technique. Hum Reprod 1998;13:1111–3.
14. Vicari E, Graziosos C, Burrello N, et al. Epididymal and testicular sperm retrieval in azoospermic patients and the outcome of intracytoplasmic sperm injection in relation to the etiology of azoospermia. Fertil Steril 2001;75:215–6.
15. Mercan R, Urman B, Alatas C, et al. Outcome of testicular sperm retrieval procedures in non-obstructive azoospermia: percutaneous aspiration versus open biopsy. Hum Reprod 2000;15:1548–51.
16. Ezeh UI, Moore HD, Cooke ID. A prospective study of multiple needle biopsies versus a single open biopsy for testicular sperm extraction in men with non-obstructive azoospermia. Hum Reprod 1998;13:3075–80.
17. Friedler S, Raziel A, Strassburger D, et al. Testicular sperm retrieval by percutaneous fine needle sperm aspiration compared with testicular sperm extraction by open biopsy in men with non-obstructive azoospermia. Hum Reprod 1997;12:1488–93.
18. Vernaeve V, Verheyen G, Goossens A, et al. How successful is repeat testicular sperm extraction in patients with azoospermia? Hum Reprod 2006;21:1551–4.
19. Schlegel PN. Testicular sperm extraction: microdissection improves sperm yield with minimal tissue excision. Hum Reprod 1999;14:131–5.
20. Amer M, Ateyah A, Hany R, et al. Prospective comparative study between microsurgical and conventional testicular sperm extraction in non-obstructive azoospermia: follow-up by serial ultrasound examinations. Hum Reprod 2000;15:653–6.
21. Okada H, Dobashi M, Yamazaki T, et al. Conventional versus microdissection testicular sperm extraction for nonobstructive azoospermia. J Urol 2002;168:1063–7.
22. Tsujimura A, Matsumiya K, Miyagawa Y, et al. Conventional multiple or microdissection testicular sperm extraction: a comparative study. Hum Reprod 2002;17:2924–9.
23. Ramasamy R, Yagan N, Schlegel PN. Structural and functional changes to the testis after conventional versus microdissection testicular sperm extraction. Urology 2005;65:1190–4.
24. Flannigan R, Bach PV, Schlegel PN. Microdissection testicular sperm extraction. Transl Androl Urol 2017;6:745–52.
25. Deruyver Y, Vanderschueren D, Van der Aa F, et al. Outcome of microdissection TESE compared to conventional TESE in non-obstructive azoospermia: a systematic review. Andrology 2014;2:20–4.
26. Bernie AM, Mata DA, Ramasamy R, et al. Comparison of microdissection testicular sperm extraction, conventional testicular sperm extraction, and testicular sperm aspiration for nonobstructive azoospermia: a systematic review and meta-analysis. Fertil Steril 2015;104:1099–103.

27. Ishikawa T, Nose R, Yamaguchi K, et al. Learning curves of microdissection testicular sperm extraction for non-obstructive azoospermia. Fertil Steril 2010;94:1008–11.
28. Schlegel PN, Su L. Physiological consequences of testicular sperm extraction. Hum Reprod 1997;12: 1688–92.
29. Harrington TG, Schauer D, Gilbert BR. Percutaneous testis biopsy: an alternative to open testicular biopsy in the evaluation of the subfertile man. J Urol 1996;156:1647–51.
30. Takada S, Tsujimura A, Ueda T, et al. Androgen decline in patients with nonobstructive azoospemia after microdissection testicular sperm extraction. Urology 2008;72:114–8.
31. Binsaleh S, Alhajeri D, Madbouly K. Microdissection testicular sperm extraction in men with nonobstructive azoospermia: experience of King Saud University Medical City, Riyadh, Saudi Arabia. Urol Ann 2017;9:136–40.
32. Eliveld J, van Wely M, Meibner A, et al. The risk of TESE-induced hypogonadism: a systematic review and meta-analysis. Hum Reprod Update 2018;24: 442–54.
33. Arïdoğan IA, Bayazït Y, Yaman M, et al. Comparison of fine-needle aspiration and open biopsy of testis in sperm retrieval and histopathologic diagnosis. Andrologia 2003;35:121–5.
34. Mahajan AD, Ali NI, Walwalkar SJ, et al. The role of fine-needle aspiration cytology of the testis in the diagnostic evaluation of infertility. BJU Int 1999;84: 485–8.
35. Qublan HS, Al-Jader KM, Al-Kaisi NS, et al. Fine needle aspiration cytology compared with open biopsy histology for the diagnosis of azoospermia. J Obstet Gynaecol 2002;22:527–31.
36. Meng MV, Cha I, Ljung B-M, et al. Testicular fine-needle aspiration in infertile men: correlation of cytologic pattern with biopsy histology. Am J Surg Pathol 2001;25:71–9.
37. Turek PJ, Ljung B-M, Cha I, et al. Diagnostic findings from testis fine needle aspiration mapping in obstructed and nonobstructed azoospermic men. J Urol 2000;163:1709–16.
38. Meng MV, Cha I, Ljung BM, et al. Relationship between classic histological pattern and sperm findings on fine needle aspiration map in infertile men. Hum Reprod 2000;15:1973–7.
39. Turek PJ, Givens CR, Schriock ED, et al. Testis sperm extraction and intracytoplasmic sperm injection guided by prior fine-needle aspiration mapping in patients with nonobstructive azoospermia. Fertil Steril 1999;71:552–7.
40. Lewin A, Reubinoff B, Porat-Katz A, et al. Testicular fine needle aspiration: the alternative method for sperm retrieval in non-obstructive azoospermia. Hum Reprod 1999;14:1785–90.
41. Jad AM, Turek PJ. Experience with testis FNA mapping and microdissection (M & M) in difficult nonobstructive azoospermia cases. Fertil Steril 2002;78:S71.
42. Jarvis S, Yee HK, Thomas N, et al. Sperm fine-needle aspiration (FNA) mapping after failed microdissection testicular sperm extraction (TESE): location and patterns of found sperm. Asian J Androl 2019;21:50–5.
43. Talas H, Yaman O, Aydos K. Outcome of repeated micro-surgical testicular sperm extraction in patients with non-obstructive azoospermia. Asian J Androl 2007;9:668–73.
44. Morris S, Yap T, Alkematy K, et al. Is there a role for salvage or redo micro-dissection testicular sperm extraction in non-obstructive azoospermia? Proceedings of the American Urologic Association. San Francisco, CA, May 18–21, 2018. Available at: https://www.auajournals.org/doi/10.1016/j.juro.2018.02.221.
45. Westlander G, Ekerhovd E, Granberg S, et al. Serial ultrasonography, hormonal profile and antisperm antibody response after testicular sperm aspiration. Hum Reprod 2001;16:2621–7.
46. Carpi A, Menchini F, Palego P, et al. Fine-needle and large-needle percutaneous aspiration biopsy of testicles in men with nonobstructive azoospermia: safety and diagnostic performance. Fertil Steril 2005;83:1029–33.
47. Chen T, Ahn J, Johnsen N, et al. Cost-effectiveness of initial fine needle aspiration mapping versus microscopic testicular sperm extraction for men with nonobstructive azoospermia. Proceedings of the American Urologic Association. Chicago, IL, May 3–6, 2019. Available at: https://www.auajournals.org/doi/10.1097/01.JU.0000556131.90620.bb.

High Sperm DNA Damage
Does Testicular Sperm Make Sense?

Keith Jarvi, MD, FRCSC

KEYWORDS

• Sperm DNA integrity • In vitro fertilization • Sperm selection • Prospective cohort study
• Live birth rates • Pregnancy rates • Testicular sperm retrieval

KEY POINTS

- High sperm DNA damage increases the risks of pregnancy loss.
- Testicular sperm have less DNA damage than sperm in the ejaculate.
- Using testicular sperm for in vitro fertilization for men with high levels of sperm DNA damage is widely used.
- Presently, there is insufficient evidence to conclude that the use of testicular sperm increases live birth rates compared with ejaculated sperm for men with high levels of sperm DNA damage.
- The use of testicular sperm retrieval for in vitro fertilization to manage men with high sperm DNA damage is not supported by the literature published to date.

BACKGROUND

In North America, approximately 15% of couples suffer from subfertility. In approximately 35% of these couples, a male factor is identified for the subfertility.[1] There are a variety of treatments available for men with subfertility, but quite often in vitro fertilization (IVF) or intra-cytoplasmic sperm insertion (ICSI) is used to help couples with male factor infertility. IVF is the process in which sperm are incubated with oocytes, whereas ICSI is the process in which individual sperm are injected directly into oocytes. Because ICSI requires the use of very few sperm and because the injection of the sperm directly into the oocyte ICSI means that the sperm do not require the ability to bind to or penetrate the oocyte, ICSI is now widely used to treat men with abnormal semen parameters, including men with low sperm counts and sperm motility, as well as for men with low numbers of morphologically normal sperm. ICSI has allowed millions of couples with infertility to become biological parents.

In North America, more than 200,000 IVF or ICSI cycles are performed yearly.[2] In Europe, there were more than 686,000 cycles performed in 2013, and in Japan, 244,000 cycles in 2015.[3,4] If a male factor is identified, more than 90% of the cycles are ICSI rather than IVF alone.[2]

The medical costs of IVF can be quite high but vary substantially by country. Chambers and colleagues[5] reported that the cost of an IVF cycle (in 2006 US$) ranged from $12,513 in the United States to $3956 in Japan. In addition, a significant amount of time and effort is taken by the couples undergoing the fertility treatments, with multiple visits to the infertility units for investigations and treatments.

Reported first in 1992 by Palermo and colleagues,[6] the use of ICSI has certainly revolutionized the treatment of male factor infertility. This group reported that ICSI bypassed the natural selection process, allowing for high fertilization, pregnancy, and live birth rates for couples with infertility, with the success rates being independent of the sperm count, motility, or morphology.[7] Other groups subsequently reported clinical studies that ICSI fertilization and pregnancy rates

Division of Urology, Department of Surgery, Institute of Medical Science, University of Toronto, Lunenfeld-Tannenbaum Research Institute, Mount Sinai Hospital, 60 Murray Street, 6th Floor, Box 19, Toronto, Ontario M5T 3L9, Canada
E-mail address: keith.jarvi@sinaihealth.ca

Urol Clin N Am 47 (2020) 165–174
https://doi.org/10.1016/j.ucl.2019.12.009

were not affected by sperm counts, motility, morphology, or even the source of the sperm (ejaculated vs epididymal) as long as the sperm were alive.[8–10]

This optimism that ICSI outcomes were independent of sperm parameters has been challenged by more recent studies showing reduced pregnancy rates and live birth rates for couples with male factor infertility. Strassburger and colleagues[11] in 2000 reported lower fertilization and pregnancy rates as well as lower live birth rates if the men had lower sperm counts, and De Vos and colleagues[12] in 2003 noted higher pregnancy rates when morphologically normal sperm were used for ICSI.

Although routine semen testing measures the sperm count, motility, and morphology, other tests of sperm function/capacity have been developed: some of the most widely used approaches are assays to measure the sperm DNA integrity (**Fig. 1**). The most common tests in use are the sperm chromatin structure assay, the sperm chromatin dispersion test, the COMET assay (**Fig. 2**), and the TUNEL assay (terminal deoxynucleotidyl transferase dUTP nick end-labeling assay).[13] Unfortunately, there is no standardized approach to the measure of sperm DNA damage, and reports on sperm DNA damage are typically a numeric value that is then interpreted as a binomial result (either high or normal/low levels of DNA fragmentation). With such a variety of different measures and normal reported ranges of sperm DNA damage, it is difficult to interpret different studies using sperm DNA damage levels as a metric.

Sperm DNA damage may occur during spermatogenesis with the induction of apoptosis (reviewed by Sakkas and Alvarez[14] in 2010), during spermiogenesis[15] (during chromatin remodeling), or posttesticular with damage owing to reactive oxygen species,[16,17] reduced seminal antioxidants,[18] and exposure to environmental/lifestyle factors, such as pollution, cigarette smoking, chemotherapies, advanced age, and some drugs.[19–21]

Impact of High Sperm DNA Damage on Intracytoplasmic Sperm Insertion Outcomes

There is now quite compelling evidence that elevated rates of sperm DNA fragmentation are associated with compromised ICSI outcomes. In a metaanalysis in 2008, Collins and colleagues[22] found an association between sperm DNA fragmentation as measured by standard sperm DNA integrity assays and pregnancy rate (odds ratio [OR] 1.44: 95% confidence interval [CI] 1.03–2.03) with ICSI, whereas Zini and colleagues[23] in 2008 noted that sperm DNA fragmentation was predictive of pregnancy loss following IVF/ICSI cycles (OR 2.48: 95% CI 1.43–5.2). Zhao and colleagues[24] in 2014 in an updated metaanalysis confirmed the above findings and noted that abnormally high levels of sperm DNA fragmentation was associated with higher pregnancy loss rates following IVF/ICSI (OR 2.68: 95% CI 1.40–5.14).

How frequently is high sperm DNA fragmentation found?

There are several studies reporting on the frequency of high sperm DNA fragmentation with reported rates up to 40% of infertile men,[25] but the author's series from Toronto found the rates of high sperm DNA fragmentation depended on the diagnosis, with high sperm DNA fragmentation found in 48% of men with bacteriospermia, 30% of men with varicoceles, and 22% of the men with idiopathic infertility.[26] Only 8% of fertile men in the series by Zini and colleagues[27] were found to have significant sperm DNA fragmentation.

How to treat men to reduce sperm DNA fragmentation?

There are potentially reversible causes for high sperm DNA fragmentation, including varicoceles, infections, and smoking.[28] A recent metaanalysis showed that varicocelectomy reduces sperm DNA fragmentation rates by −3.37% (95% CI: −4.09 to −2.65).[29] Smoking has long been associated with male infertility, but the negative impact of smoking on sperm DNA fragmentation has only more recently been reported.[30–32] Although smoking cessation is recommended, the impact of cessation on sperm DNA has not been reported. Infections and inflammations of the male reproductive tract may also be related to sperm DNA fragmentation, with improvements in DNA integrity with specific therapies.[33–35] For most men, no potentially reversible causes are identified. These men have been treated with antioxidants with evidence of a significant reduction of sperm DNA fragmentation (reviewed by Zini and colleagues[36] and Showell and colleagues[37]) in 1 metaanalysis of 2 studies showing a reduction of −13.85% (95% CI: −17.85 to −10.41). Despite these therapies, many men end up with abnormally high rates of sperm DNA fragmentation, which may be contributing to IVF/ICSI failures.

If therapies to improve sperm DNA integrity are ineffective, are there alternative ways to improve the reproductive outcomes with intracytoplasmic sperm insertion for men with sperm DNA fragmentation?

It is well recognized that there is intense sperm-to-sperm variability (within the same semen specimens) in the levels of DNA fragmentation.

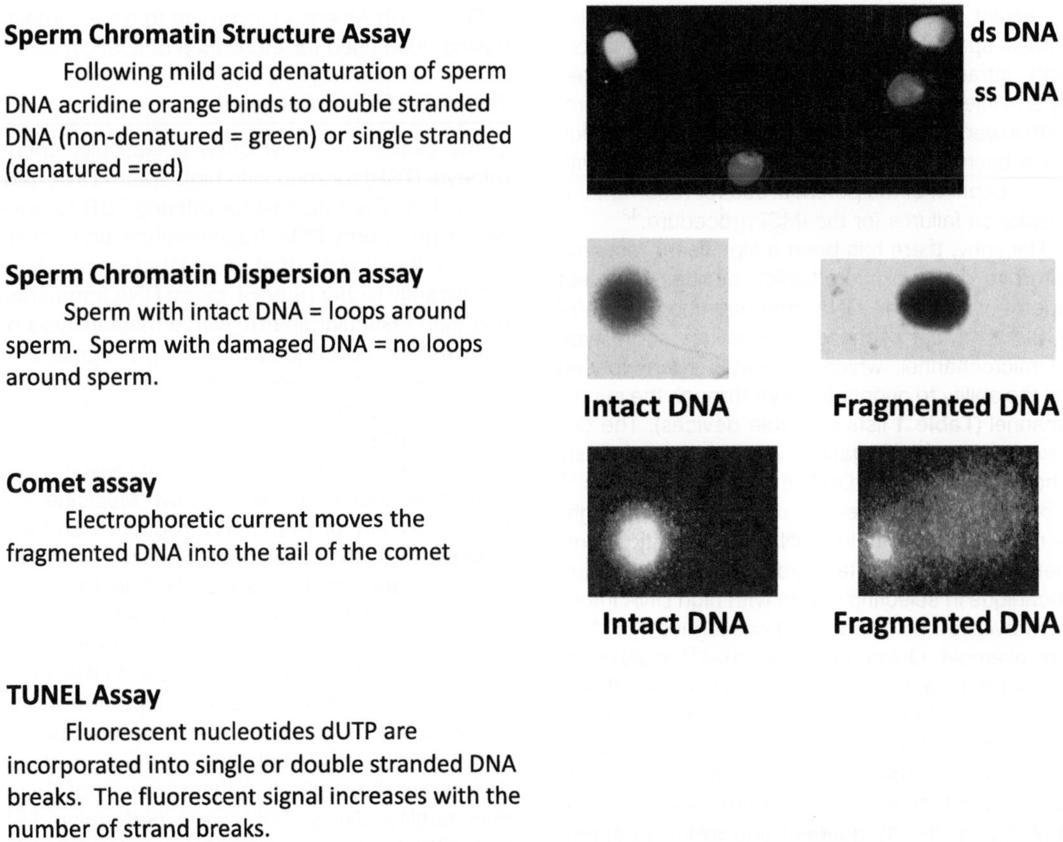
Sperm Chromatin Structure Assay
Following mild acid denaturation of sperm DNA acridine orange binds to double stranded DNA (non-denatured = green) or single stranded (denatured =red)
ds DNA
ss DNA
Sperm Chromatin Dispersion assay
Sperm with intact DNA = loops around sperm. Sperm with damaged DNA = no loops around sperm.
Intact DNA
Fragmented DNA
Comet assay
Electrophoretic current moves the fragmented DNA into the tail of the comet
Intact DNA
Fragmented DNA
TUNEL Assay
Fluorescent nucleotides dUTP are incorporated into single or double stranded DNA breaks. The fluorescent signal increases with the number of strand breaks.

Fig. 1. Commonly used assays to measure sperm DNA damage levels. dsDNA, double-stranded dsDNA; ssDNA, single-stranded DNA; TUNEL, terminal deoxynucleotidyl transferase nick end-labeling assay.

Conceptually, if there was some way to choose individual sperm with less DNA fragmentation, this method should improve the reproductive outcomes following ICSI. Unfortunately, with the present technology in use, there is no way to measure the level of DNA fragmentation in an individual sperm and then use that sperm for ICSI.

Selection of Sperm with Less DNA Damage

The standard sperm selection techniques use a combination of centrifugation of the sperm through a density gradient, often followed by a "swim-up" procedure to select highly motile sperm.[38] This process does select sperm with higher motility and with lower DNA fragmentation.[39] This technique remains the standard selection technique for most fertility centers in North America.

There have been several other different procedures used to select sperm with lower DNA fragmentation. *Hyaluronan binding* has been used to select sperm with lower DNA fragmentation rates: these sperm have subsequently been used for the ICSI procedure (PICSI technique: physiologic hyaluronan-selected intracytoplasmic sperm injection).[40] This technique has not been shown to improve live birth rates, with a very large recent study recommending that PICSI be abandoned for sperm selection.[40,41] Others have reported the use of high-resolution imaging of the sperm

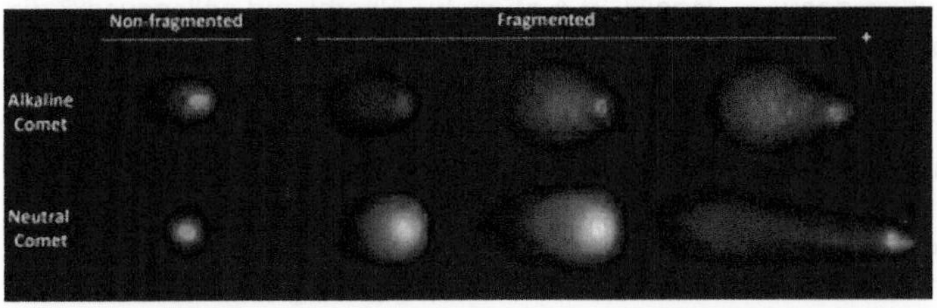

Fig. 2. Examples of Comet assays showing "high," "normal," and low sperm DNA integrity. An electrophoretic current separates the fragmented DNA into the tail of the comet, leaving the nonfragmented DNA in the head of the comet.

to select sperm with normal sperm organelles (motile sperm organelle morphology examination) and intracytoplasmic morphologically selected sperm injection (IMSI), both of which select sperm with lower DNA fragmentation but neither of which have been shown to increase live birth rates with the exception of the potential use for recurrent implantation failures for the IMSI procedure.[42]

Recently, there has been a significant research effort to develop microfluidics devices to select sperm with lower DNA fragmentation for IVF/ICSI.[43–50] Most of these devices use some type of microchannel, which separates sperm based on the ability to negotiate/swim through the microchannel (**Table 1** lists available devices). The devices avoid centrifugation, which was previously shown to increase DNA fragmentation rates.[39] Consistently, these devices are able to select highly motile sperm with low DNA fragmentation, outperforming the standard sperm selection technique in selecting sperm with high DNA integrity (reviewed by Nosrati and colleagues[47]).[44,47,51] For example, Quinn and colleagues[44] in 2018 reported that sperm selected using a microfluidic device had virtually undetectable rates of sperm DNA fragmentation as measured by the sperm chromatin dispersion assay, rates that were significantly less than the rates in sperm selected using a standard density gradient and swim-up sperm selection technique. Unfortunately, there are no data for any microfluidic device on aneuploidy rates for selected sperm. Although the microfluidic approaches look promising for the selection of sperm for IVF/ICSI, *there are no randomized controlled trials documenting improvements in reproductive outcomes using these devices*. In 2018, Yetkinel and colleagues[43] reported on a randomized controlled trial on the use of the Fertile Chip device to select sperm for ICSI outcomes compared with the standard sperm preparation technique. They reported similar fertilization, pregnancy, and live birth rates between the 2 groups. This group selected couples with unexplained infertility not based on any particular semen parameter. There is a registered clinical trial on the use of the Zymot device for couples who have had "poor embryo quality" in a previous IVF cycle, but the details of this study were not recorded at clinicaltrials.gov.

Despite the lack of well-controlled studies documenting higher live birth rates using microfluidics-selected sperm, several companies are selling these devices for use to select sperm before IVF, and 1 device (Zymot or FERTILE) is approved by the Food and Drug Administration for sale in the United States. The Zymot device is commercially available and in clinical use to select sperm for ICSI in North America (according to Koek Biotech, having been used for thousands of ICSI cycles).

Testicular Sperm Retrieval

Some centers are now offering testicular sperm retrieval (TSR) for men with high sperm DNA fragmentation. The rationale for offering TSR for men with high sperm DNA fragmentation undergoing ICSI is the finding that ejaculated sperm have significantly higher rates of sperm DNA fragmentation than testicular sperm, with a metaanalysis by Esteves and colleagues[52] showing a significantly lower sperm DNA fragmentation rate in testicular versus ejaculated sperm (8.9% ± 5.1% vs 33.4% ± 12.8%).[53,54]

Presently, none of the major fertility associations (American Society of Reproductive Medicine, European Society of Human Reproductive Endocrinology, and the Canadian Fertility Andrology Society) supports the use of TSR to treat men with high sperm DNA damage. In fact, the American Society of Reproductive Medicine does not even support the routine use of sperm DNA integrity testing.[55] Despite the lack of support from the major fertility associations, this procedure is now being offered in an unknown number of clinics throughout the world. In a recent survey of Canadian fertility clinics, 70% were performing TSR with ICSI for nonazoospermic men (reported by Zini and colleagues[56]).

Comparing Testicular Sperm Retrieval Versus Ejaculated Sperm Reproductive Outcomes with Intracytoplasmic Sperm Insertion

Although the evidence that sperm DNA damage is less in the TSR sperm than in the ejaculate is compelling, what evidence exists to support the use of TSR to improve live birth rates for men with high sperm DNA damage using ICSI? Greco and colleagues[54] were the first to report higher pregnancy rates in testicular versus ejaculated sperm for those with high sperm DNA fragmentation, with the reported pregnancy rate of 44% in the TSR group versus 6% in the ejaculated sperm group. Over the years, there has been a series of other noncontrolled studies showing improved pregnancy rates with TSR compared with ejaculated sperm for men with high sperm DNA damage.[57–64] A study by Alharbi and colleagues[65] did not identify increased live birth rates.

In the metaanalysis by Esteves and colleagues[52] reported in 2017, it was found that ICSI using testicular sperm compared with ejaculated sperm resulted in lower fertilization rates (59.8% vs 68.7%, $P<.001$), higher clinical pregnancies (50% vs 29.4%, $P<.001$), and higher live birth rates

Table 1
Microfluidic devices being marketed

Device	Selection Mode	% DNA Fragmentation Index		Concentration (Selected/Raw)	Clinical (IVF/ICSI) Trial/Countries	IVF/ICSI Test Results	Reference/Web Site
		Raw	Selected				
FERTILE	3D swimming	31–40	0–0.2	0.28	In progress/ United States, Turkey	• Pregnancy %: 34% when chip is used vs 23% with Percoll method (performed in Turkey)	• Quinn et al, 2018[72] • http://www.koekbiotech.com
QUALIS	3D swimming	N/A	0–9	0.08	Japan	• No information available	• cho et al, 2003[73] • http://www.menicon-lifescience.com
ZECH SELECTOR 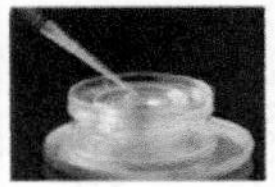	3D swimming	5–42.1	0–2.5	N/A	No information available	• No information available	• Seiringer et al, 2013[74] • https//www.kinderwunsuch.at/de/zech-selector.com
CS10	Electrophoretic separation	16	5	0.18	Australia	• No significant difference in fertilization compared with density-gradient centrifugation (62.4% vs 63.6%)	• Fleming et al, 2008[75] • http://www.memphasys.com.au/
Seaforia 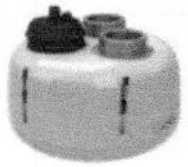	Thermotaxis+ 3D swimming	N/A	N/A	0.20	Australia	• No information available	• Irving et al, 2013[76] • http://wwwlotusbio.com

Abbreviation: N/A, not applicable.

(46.9% vs 25.6%, $P<.001$) with an OR of 2.58 (95% CI: 1.54–4.35). However, the study was limited with the included reports being noncontrolled, in some cases comparing ICSI outcomes sequentially for the same couple and only a total of 2 studies reported live birth rates. As previously reported by Khan and colleagues[66] in 1996, these types of crossover studies lead to significant overestimation of pregnancy rates. In addition, data used in the metaanalysis included a study in which the sperm had been cryopreserved without a subanalysis of the effect of cryopreservation on the reproductive outcomes.[63]

Awaga and colleagues[67] in 2018 performed a systematic review on the use of testicular sperm for men without azoospermia and identified a total of 4 studies eligible for the review, with only 2 studies specifically on the use of TSR for high sperm DNA damage. Because of the population heterogeneity, a metaanalysis was not feasible, so the investigators performed a systematic review. The invstigators' conclusion was that the existing studies were too heterogeneous to compare and that the data did not support the use of TSR to manage men with high sperm DNA damage.

What Are the Risks Associated with Testicular Sperm Retrieval?

There are risks associated with the biopsy and even potentially the use of testicular sperm. Esteves and colleagues[61] reported a surgical complication rate of 6.2%, although this included no significant complications. In the author's unpublished series (Jarvi and Lo, 2014) following 50 men after a testis biopsy, there were no significant complications and only 1/50 had an intratesticular hematoma documented by ultrasound that resolved spontaneously. The author's series also has evidence that testicular sperm aneuploidy rates are significantly higher than ejaculated sperm aneuploidy rates. Moskovtsev and colleagues[68] reported that although sperm DNA fragmentation rates were lower in testicular versus ejaculated sperm (14.9% $\pm$ 5.0% vs 40.6% $\pm$ 14.8%, $P<.05$), the aneuploidy rates for 5 analyzed chromosomes using fluorescent in situ hybridization were significantly higher in the testicular sperm (12.41% $\pm$ 3.7% vs 5.77% $\pm$ 1.2%, $P<.05$). The group suggested that the apparent advantage of lower sperm DNA damage in the testicular sperm may be offset by the disadvantage of higher aneuploidy rates. However, Cheung and colleagues[64] in 2019 reviewed their results prospectively comparing sperm DNA aneuploidy rates measured by whole-exome sequencing in ejaculated versus testicular sperm, finding that the testicular sperm did not have significantly different aneuploidy rates.

What Are the Potential Cost Advantages of Testicular Sperm Retrieval for Men with High Sperm DNA Damage?

For this calculation, assume that the metaanalysis of Esteves and colleagues[52] provides accurate estimates of the effect size of TSR on live birth rates; then, a cost/live birth can be calculated (biopsy costs \$1250–\$2500 in Canada based on fees paid in Montreal and Toronto, IVF cost US\$ \$12,513 in 2006; **Table 2**).

For individual patients and payers, this is a potential significant saving. Considering that 22% of men with idiopathic infertility have high rates of sperm DNA damage, if TSR actually results in higher pregnancy rates, there would be a significant impact on payers if TSR was adopted.

What Is Required to Further Study the Role of Testicular Sperm Retrieval in the Management of Men with High Sperm DNA Damage?

Presently, the reports available do not provide adequate evidence to support the use of TSR to manage men with high sperm DNA damage. However, the relatively low risk associated with the TSR procedure, the available studies that suggest a possible positive effect on live birth rates, and the lack of a viable proven alternative to improve pregnancy rates for men with high sperm DNA damage all lead to the obvious conclusion, that further studies are needed in the area before concluding that TSR should be a standard approach to manage men with high levels of sperm DNA damage.

There are several issues that need to be addressed: a lack of a standard technique to

Table 2
Cost per live birth for testicular versus ejaculated sperm used for intracytoplasmic sperm insertion for men with high sperm DNA damage

	Biopsy, $	IVF Direct Cost, $	Live Birth Rate	Cost/Live Birth, $	Saving/Live Birth, $
Ejaculated sperm	—	12,513	0.256	48,878	—
Testicular sperm	1875	12,513	0.469	30,678	18,200

measure sperm DNA damage levels and a lack of standard normal range values limit the ability to compare studies of sperm DNA damage.[13] Second, the standard reports on sperm DNA damage are categorical (reported as either high or normal/low), whereas the numerical value does provide added information on prognosis. Although a cutoff value for DNA damage is useful to provide guidance on the choice of assisted reproductive technologies (Spano and colleagues[69] using a cutoff value to predict the need for IVF or ICSI), it has become clear that very high rates of sperm DNA damage have different ICSI success rates than those with marginally elevated rates of sperm DNA damage.[70]

Complicating this, a controlled trial to definitively answer the question about the role of TSR for men with high sperm DNA damage would be ideal, but difficult, because recruitment would be challenging.[71]

SUMMARY

High levels of sperm DNA fragmentation lead to poorer reproductive outcomes, with lower pregnancy and live birth rates following IVF and ICSI. There is active research on techniques to select sperm from the semen with the least DNA damage, but presently, none of the techniques has been proven to increase live birth rates. An alternative has been to retrieve sperm from the testicle. The sperm in the testicles has not been exposed to the more hostile environment of the epididymis/vas deferens and has less DNA damage than ejaculated sperm. Many fertility centers offer this sperm retrieval procedure for men with high ejaculated sperm DNA damage, despite this procedure not being supported by the major fertility organizations. The existing studies on the use of sperm retrieval in this setting are single-center, prospective, noncontrolled studies and do not provide adequate evidence to support the use of sperm retrieval to treat men with high levels of ejaculated sperm DNA damage. Further studies are required before the acceptance of TSR for high sperm DNA damage as a standard of care.

DISCLOSURE

The authors have nothing to disclose. There is no funding to support this research.

REFERENCES

1. Stern JE, Brown MB, Wantman E, et al. Live birth rates and birth outcomes by diagnosis using linked cycles from the SART CORS database. J Assist Reprod Genet 2013;30(11):1445–50.
2. Sunderam S, Kissin DM, Crawford SB, et al. Assisted reproductive technology surveillance–United States, 2014. MMWR Surveill Summ 2017;66(6):1–24.
3. European IVF-monitoring Consortium (EIM), European Society of Human Reproduction and Embryology (ESHRE), Calhaz-Jorge C, et al. Assisted reproductive technology in Europe, 2013: results generated from European registers by ESHRE. Hum Reprod 2017;32(10):1957–73.
4. Saito H, Jwa SC, Kuwahara A, et al. Assisted reproductive technology in Japan: a summary report for 2015 by the Ethics Committee of the Japan Society of Obstetrics and Gynecology. Reprod Med Biol 2018;17(1):20–8.
5. Chambers GM, Sullivan EA, Ishihara O, et al. The economic impact of assisted reproductive technology: a review of selected developed countries. Fertil Steril 2009;91(6):2281–94.
6. Palermo G, Joris H, Devroey P, et al. Pregnancies after intracytoplasmic injection of single spermatozoon into an oocyte. Lancet 1992;340(8810):17–8.
7. Palermo G, Joris H, Derde MP, et al. Sperm characteristics and outcome of human assisted fertilization by subzonal insemination and intracytoplasmic sperm injection. Fertil Steril 1993;59(4):826–35.
8. Mansour RT, Aboulghar MA, Serour GI, et al. The effect of sperm parameters on the outcome of intracytoplasmic sperm injection. Fertil Steril 1995;64(5):982–6.
9. Silber SJ, Van Steirteghem AC, Liu J, et al. High fertilization and pregnancy rate after intracytoplasmic sperm injection with spermatozoa obtained from testicle biopsy. Hum Reprod 1995;10(1):148–52.
10. Nagy ZP, Liu J, Joris H, et al. The result of intracytoplasmic sperm injection is not related to any of the three basic sperm parameters. Hum Reprod 1995;10(5):1123–9.
11. Strassburger D, Friedler S, Raziel A, et al. Very low sperm count affects the result of intracytoplasmic sperm injection. J Assist Reprod Genet 2000;17(8):431–6.
12. De Vos A, Van De Velde H, Joris H, et al. Influence of individual sperm morphology on fertilization, embryo morphology, and pregnancy outcome of intracytoplasmic sperm injection. Fertil Steril 2003;79(1):42–8.
13. Agarwal A, Majzoub A, Esteves SC, et al. Clinical utility of sperm DNA fragmentation testing: practice recommendations based on clinical scenarios. Transl Androl Urol 2016;5(6):935–50.
14. Sakkas D, Alvarez JG. Sperm DNA fragmentation: mechanisms of origin, impact on reproductive outcome, and analysis. Fertil Steril 2010;93(4):1027–36.

15. McPherson SM, Longo FJ. Nicking of rat spermatid and spermatozoa DNA: possible involvement of DNA topoisomerase II. Dev Biol 1993;158(1):122–30.
16. Ollero M, Gil-Guzman E, Lopez MC, et al. Characterization of subsets of human spermatozoa at different stages of maturation: implications in the diagnosis and treatment of male infertility. Hum Reprod 2001;16(9):1912–21.
17. Lopes S, Jurisicova A, Sun JG, et al. Reactive oxygen species: potential cause for DNA fragmentation in human spermatozoa. Hum Reprod 1998;13(4):896–900.
18. Shamsi MB, Venkatesh S, Kumar R, et al. Antioxidant levels in blood and seminal plasma and their impact on sperm parameters in infertile men. Indian J Biochem Biophys 2010;47(1):38–43.
19. Sharma R, Biedenharn KR, Fedor JM, et al. Lifestyle factors and reproductive health: taking control of your fertility. Reprod Biol Endocrinol 2013;11:66.
20. Sharma R, Harlev A, Agarwal A, et al. Cigarette smoking and semen quality: a new meta-analysis examining the effect of the 2010 World Health Organization laboratory methods for the examination of human semen. Eur Urol 2016;70(4):635–45.
21. Rubes J, Selevan SG, Evenson DP, et al. Episodic air pollution is associated with increased DNA fragmentation in human sperm without other changes in semen quality. Hum Reprod 2005;20(10):2776–83.
22. Collins JA, Barnhart KT, Schlegel PN. Do sperm DNA integrity tests predict pregnancy with in vitro fertilization? Fertil Steril 2008;89(4):823–31.
23. Zini A, Boman JM, Belzile E, et al. Sperm DNA damage is associated with an increased risk of pregnancy loss after IVF and ICSI: systematic review and meta-analysis. Hum Reprod 2008;23(12):2663–8.
24. Zhao J, Zhang Q, Wang Y, et al. Whether sperm deoxyribonucleic acid fragmentation has an effect on pregnancy and miscarriage after in vitro fertilization/intracytoplasmic sperm injection: a systematic review and meta-analysis. Fertil Steril 2014;102(4):998–1005.e8.
25. Simon L, Proutski I, Stevenson M, et al. Sperm DNA damage has a negative association with live-birth rates after IVF. Reprod Biomed Online 2013;26(1):68–78.
26. Moskovtsev SI, Mullen JB, Lecker I, et al. Frequency and severity of sperm DNA damage in patients with confirmed cases of male infertility of different aetiologies. Reprod Biomed Online 2010;20(6):759–63.
27. Zini A, Fischer MA, Sharir S, et al. Prevalence of abnormal sperm DNA denaturation in fertile and infertile men. Urology 2002;60(6):1069–72.
28. Zini A, Dohle G. Are varicoceles associated with increased deoxyribonucleic acid fragmentation? Fertil Steril 2011;96(6):1283–7.
29. Wang YJ, Zhang RQ, Lin YJ, et al. Relationship between varicocele and sperm DNA damage and the effect of varicocele repair: a meta-analysis. Reprod Biomed Online 2012;25(3):307–14.
30. Gavriliouk D, Aitken RJ. Damage to sperm DNA mediated by reactive oxygen species: its impact on human reproduction and the health trajectory of offspring. Adv Exp Med Biol 2015;868:23–47.
31. Agarwal A, Prabakaran SA. Mechanism, measurement, and prevention of oxidative stress in male reproductive physiology. Indian J Exp Biol 2005;43(11):963–74.
32. Dai JB, Wang ZX, Qiao ZD. The hazardous effects of tobacco smoking on male fertility. Asian J Androl 2015;17(6):954–60.
33. Aitken RJ, Baker MA. Oxidative stress, spermatozoa and leukocytic infiltration: relationships forged by the opposing forces of microbial invasion and the search for perfection. J Reprod Immunol 2013;100(1):11–9.
34. Pourmasumi S, Sabeti P, Rahiminia T, et al. The etiologies of DNA abnormalities in male infertility: an assessment and review. Int J Reprod Biomed (Yazd) 2017;15(6):331–44.
35. Moskovtsev SI, Lecker I, Mullen JB, et al. Cause-specific treatment in patients with high sperm DNA damage resulted in significant DNA improvement. Syst Biol Reprod Med 2009;55(2):109–15.
36. Zini A, San Gabriel M, Baazeem A. Antioxidants and sperm DNA damage: a clinical perspective. J Assist Reprod Genet 2009;26(8):427–32.
37. Showell MG, Mackenzie-Proctor R, Brown J, et al. Antioxidants for male subfertility. Cochrane Database Syst Rev 2014;(12):CD007411.
38. World Health Organization DoRHaR. WHO laboratory manual for the examination and processing of human semen. 5th ed: WHO; 2010.
39. Zini A, Finelli A, Phang D, et al. Influence of semen processing technique on human sperm DNA integrity. Urology 2000;56(6):1081–4.
40. Miller D, Pavitt S, Sharma V, et al. Physiological, hyaluronan-selected intracytoplasmic sperm injection for infertility treatment (HABSelect): a parallel, two-group, randomised trial. Lancet 2019;393(10170):416–22.
41. Kirkman-Brown J, Pavitt S, Khalaf Y, et al. Sperm selection for assisted reproduction by prior hyaluronan binding: the HABSelect RCT 2019. Southampton (UK) NIHR Journals Library.
42. Boitrelle F, Guthauser B, Alter L, et al. High-magnification selection of spermatozoa prior to oocyte injection: confirmed and potential indications. Reprod Biomed Online 2014;28(1):6–13.
43. Yetkinel S, Kilicdag EB, Aytac PC, et al. Effects of the microfluidic chip technique in sperm selection

for intracytoplasmic sperm injection for unexplained infertility: a prospective, randomized controlled trial. J Assist Reprod Genet 2019;36(3):403–9.
44. Quinn MM, Jalalian L, Ribeiro S, et al. Microfluidic sorting selects sperm for clinical use with reduced DNA damage compared to density gradient centrifugation with swim-up in split semen samples. Hum Reprod 2018. https://doi.org/10.1093/humrep/dey239.
45. Bhagwat S, Sontakke S, K D, et al. Chemotactic behavior of spermatozoa captured using a microfluidic chip. Biomicrofluidics 2018;12(2):024112.
46. Avalos-Duran G, Canedo-Del Angel AME, Rivero-Murillo J, et al. Physiological ICSI (PICSI) vs. conventional ICSI in couples with male factor: a systematic review. JBRA Assist Reprod 2018;22(2):139–47.
47. Nosrati R, Graham PJ, Zhang B, et al. Microfluidics for sperm analysis and selection. Nat Rev Urol 2017;14(12):707–30.
48. Lohinova O, Pitko V, Sinilo N, et al. Comparative analysis of sperm selection methods before the intra cytoplasmic sperm injection procedure. Georgian Med News 2017;(271):7–11.
49. Nosrati R, Driouchi A, Yip CM, et al. Two-dimensional slither swimming of sperm within a micrometre of a surface. Nat Commun 2015;6:8703.
50. Nosrati R, Vollmer M, Eamer L, et al. Rapid selection of sperm with high DNA integrity. Lab Chip 2014; 14(6):1142–50.
51. Ko YJ, Maeng JH, Hwang SY, et al. Design, fabrication, and testing of a microfluidic device for thermotaxis and chemotaxis assays of sperm. SLAS technology 2018;23(6):507–15.
52. Esteves SC, Roque M, Bradley CK, et al. Reproductive outcomes of testicular versus ejaculated sperm for intracytoplasmic sperm injection among men with high levels of DNA fragmentation in semen: systematic review and meta-analysis. Fertil Steril 2017; 108(3):456–67.e1.
53. Moskovtsev SI, Jarvi K, Mullen JB, et al. Testicular spermatozoa have statistically significantly lower DNA damage compared with ejaculated spermatozoa in patients with unsuccessful oral antioxidant treatment. Fertil Steril 2010;93(4):1142–6.
54. Greco E, Scarselli F, Iacobelli M, et al. Efficient treatment of infertility due to sperm DNA damage by ICSI with testicular spermatozoa. Hum Reprod 2005; 20(1):226–30.
55. Practice Committee of the American Society for Reproductive Medicine. The clinical utility of sperm DNA integrity testing: a guideline. Fertil Steril 2013; 99(3):673–7.
56. Zini A, Bach PV, Al-Malki AH, et al. Use of testicular sperm for ICSI in oligozoospermic couples: how far should we go? Hum Reprod 2017;32(1):7–13.
57. Arafa M, AlMalki A, AlBadr M, et al. ICSI outcome in patients with high DNA fragmentation: testicular versus ejaculated spermatozoa. Andrologia 2018; 50(1). https://doi.org/10.1111/and.12835.
58. Zhang J, Xue H, Qiu F, et al. Testicular spermatozoon is superior to ejaculated spermatozoon for intracytoplasmic sperm injection to achieve pregnancy in infertile males with high sperm DNA damage. Andrologia 2019;51(2):e13175.
59. Pabuccu EG, Caglar GS, Tangal S, et al. Testicular versus ejaculated spermatozoa in ICSI cycles of normozoospermic men with high sperm DNA fragmentation and previous ART failures. Andrologia 2017; 49(2). https://doi.org/10.1111/and.12609.
60. Hayden RP, Wright DL, Toth TL, et al. Selective use of percutaneous testis biopsy to optimize IVF-ICSI outcomes: a case series. Fertil Res Pract 2016;2:7.
61. Esteves SC, Sanchez-Martin F, Sanchez-Martin P, et al. Comparison of reproductive outcome in oligozoospermic men with high sperm DNA fragmentation undergoing intracytoplasmic sperm injection with ejaculated and testicular sperm. Fertil Steril 2015;104(6):1398–405.
62. Mehta A, Bolyakov A, Schlegel PN, et al. Higher pregnancy rates using testicular sperm in men with severe oligospermia. Fertil Steril 2015;104(6): 1382–7.
63. Bradley CK, McArthur SJ, Gee AJ, et al. Intervention improves assisted conception intracytoplasmic sperm injection outcomes for patients with high levels of sperm DNA fragmentation: a retrospective analysis. Andrology 2016;4(5):903–10.
64. Cheung S, Schlegel PN, Rosenwaks Z, et al. Revisiting aneuploidy profile of surgically retrieved spermatozoa by whole exome sequencing molecular karyotype. PLoS One 2019;14(1):e0210079.
65. Alharbi M, Hamouche F, Phillips S, et al. Use of testicular sperm in couples with SCSA-defined high sperm DNA fragmentation and failed intracytoplasmic sperm injection using ejaculated sperm. Asian J Androl 2019. https://doi.org/10.4103/aja.aja_99_19.
66. Khan KS, Daya S, Collins JA, et al. Empirical evidence of bias in infertility research: overestimation of treatment effect in crossover trials using pregnancy as the outcome measure. Fertil Steril 1996; 65(5):939–45.
67. Awaga HA, Bosdou JK, Goulis DG, et al. Testicular versus ejaculated spermatozoa for ICSI in patients without azoospermia: a systematic review. Reprod Biomed Online 2018;37(5):573–80.
68. Moskovtsev SI, Alladin N, Lo KC, et al. A comparison of ejaculated and testicular spermatozoa aneuploidy rates in patients with high sperm DNA damage. Syst Biol Reprod Med 2012;58(3):142–8.
69. Spano M, Bonde JP, Hjollund HI, et al. Sperm chromatin damage impairs human fertility. The Danish First Pregnancy Planner Study Team. Fertil Steril 2000;73(1):43–50.

70. Simon L, Lewis SE. Sperm DNA damage or progressive motility: which one is the better predictor of fertilization in vitro? Syst Biol Reprod Med 2011; 57(3):133–8.
71. Mehta A, Esteves SC, Schlegel PN, et al. Use of testicular sperm in nonazoospermic males. Fertil Steril 2018;109(6):981–7.
72. Quinn MM, Jalalian L, Ribeiro S, et al. Microfluidic sorting selects sperm for clinical use with reduced DNA damage compared to density gradient centrifugation with swim-up in split semen samples. Human Reproduction 2018;33(8):1388–93.
73. Cho BS, Schuster TG, Zhu X, et al. Passively Driven Integrated Microfluidic System for Separation of Motile Sperm. Analytical Chemistry 2003;75(7):1671–5.
74. Seiringer M, Maurer M, Shebl O, et al. Efficacy of a sperm-selection chamber in terms of morphology, aneuploidy and DNA packaging. Reproductive BioMedicine Online 2013;27(1):81–8.
75. Fleming SD, Ilad RS, Griffin A-MG, et al. Prospective controlled trial of an electrophoretic method of sperm preparation for assisted reproduction: comparison with density gradient centrifugation. Human Reproduction 2008;23(12):2646–51.
76. Irving J, Rabbitt TJ, Tooth RM, et al. Suitability of the Seaforia™ sperm separation system for use in art. Fertility and Sterility 2013;100(3):S452.

Round Spermatid Injection

Kelli X. Gross, MD[a,*], Brent M. Hanson, MD[b], James M. Hotaling, MD, FECSM[c]

KEYWORDS

• Azoospermia • Assisted reproductive technology • In vitro fertilization • Male factor infertility
• Round spermatid injection • Testicular sperm extraction

KEY POINTS

- The likelihood of successful identification of mature spermatozoa during a microdissection testicular sperm extraction procedure performed for azoospermia is between 40% and 60%.
- Round spermatids, which are immature precursors to mature spermatozoa, are seen in approximately 30% of men with nonobstructive azoospermia without sperm seen at the time of microdissection testicular sperm extraction.
- A recent publication from 2018 reported that successful births could be achieved through the use of round spermatid injection (ROSI) and that children born from ROSI were not at an increased risk for congenital malformations.
- Concerns regarding the potential risk of abnormal epigenetic patterns following ROSI remain.
- Overall low success rates have limited the clinical application of ROSI, although improvements in the identification of round spermatids and the technique itself may lead to higher utilization in the future.

INTRODUCTION

Azoospermia affects 10% to 15% of infertile men and is defined as no sperm seen in the ejaculate in a centrifuged sample.[1] Although patients with obstructive azoospermia are likely to have sperm retrieved with a procedure[2] such as a testicular sperm aspiration (TESA), around 60% of men with azoospermia have nonobstructive azoospermia (NOA) and thus lower rates of successful sperm retrieval.[3] NOA is due to defects in spermatogenesis, usually from primary testicular dysfunction.[4] Studies have shown that the likelihood of retrieval of sperm in NOA patients during microdissection testicular sperm extraction (microTESE), the standard of care for sperm extraction in men with NOA, is between 40% and 60%.[5,6] Y-chromosome microdeletion is present in 3% to 15% of men with severe oligozoospermia as well as in men with NOA.[7] In a sizable portion of azoospermic men, there is no sperm seen after microTESE, making it impossible for these men to father biologic offspring. Round spermatids are precursors of mature spermatozoa and are seen in about 30% of NOA men with no spermatozoa seen on microTESE[8] (**Fig. 1**). These are immature sperm cells that still contain a haploid genome, similar to the genetic composition of mature spermatozoa. Round spermatid injection (ROSI) uses this fact to inject these sperm precursors directly into an oocyte in hopes of fertilization and pregnancy.

SPERMATOGENESIS AND SPERM FUNCTION

Spermatogenesis is the process by which diploid spermatogonia become haploid spermatozoa (**Fig. 2**).[9] The spermatogonia increase in number via mitosis, and in the first stage of spermatogenesis, mitotic division results in diploid primary spermatocytes.[10] These primary spermatocytes undergo meiosis I to form secondary

[a] Division of Urology, Department of Surgery, University of Utah, 50 North Medical Drive, Salt Lake City, UT 84132, USA; [b] IVI-RMA New Jersey, Sidney Kimmel Medical College, Thomas Jefferson University, 140 Allen Road, Basking Ridge, NJ 07920, USA; [c] University of Utah Center for Reconstructive Urology & Men's Health, 675 Arapeen Way, Suite 205, Salt Lake City, UT 84108, USA
* Corresponding author.
E-mail address: kelli.gross@utah.edu

Urol Clin N Am 47 (2020) 175–183
https://doi.org/10.1016/j.ucl.2019.12.004
0094-0143/20/Published by Elsevier Inc.

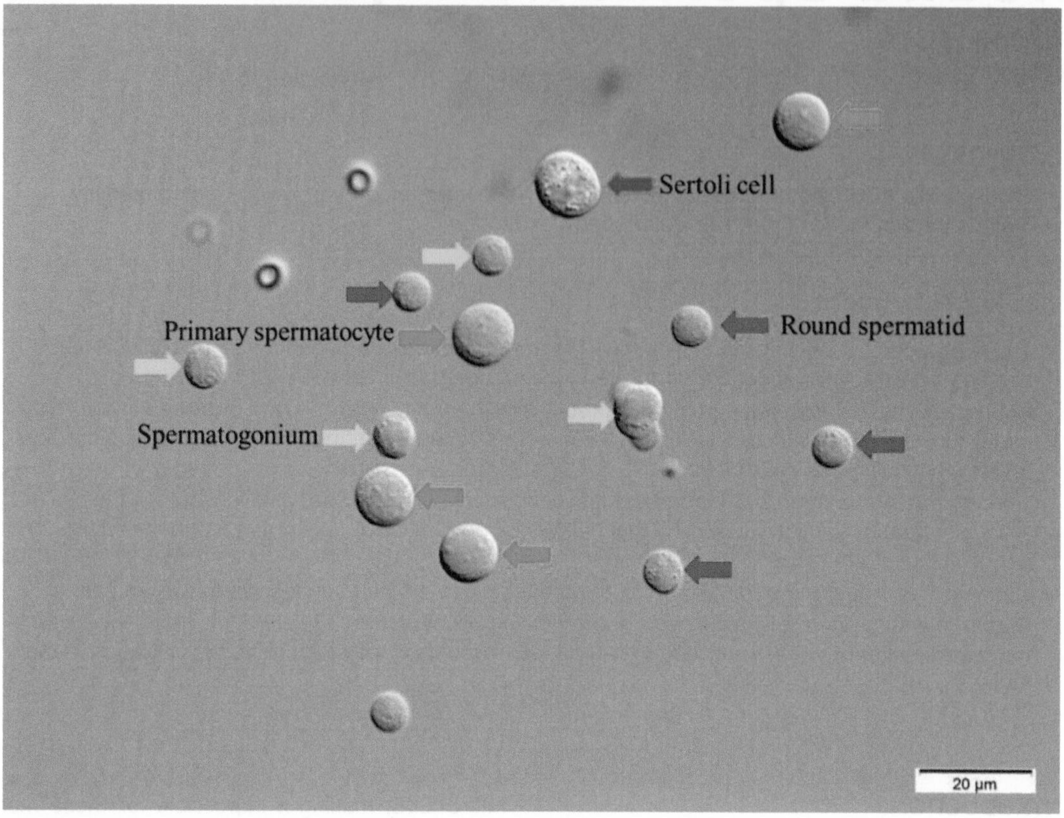

Fig. 1. Testicular cells after processing. *(Reprinted* by permission from the American Society for Reproductive Medicine [Tanaka, A., Suzuki, K., Nagayoshi, M. et al.: Ninety babies born after round spermatid injection into oocytes: survey of their development from fertilization to 2 years of age. Fertility and Sterility. 2018;110:443.])

spermatocytes and meiosis II to form spermatids,[11] such as round spermatids. At this point, spermatids have the haploid genetic material that spermatozoa contain, but the spermatids are not yet motile and are not yet able to fertilize an oocyte. In the next phase, also called spermiogenesis, the round spermatids become elongated and eventually develop a tail as they progress to become mature spermatozoa. For normal fertilization to occur, the spermatozoa must provide genetic material to the oocyte by means of the centrosome and initiate oocyte activation.[12]

HISTORY OF ASSISTED REPRODUCTION IN AZOOSPERMIA

Intracytoplasmic sperm injection (ICSI) was developed in the 1990s and has been revolutionary in allowing paternity for men with severe male factor infertility.[13–15] In this procedure, a single spermatozoon is directly injected into the oocyte. This allows for testicular sperm extraction as an assisted reproductive technology, because sperm retrieved by these methods have not fully matured and do not yet have the ability to swim or fertilize an egg. Despite initial theoretic concerns about the long-term outcomes of children born by ICSI, any negative effects appear to be minimal, and ICSI has seen widespread use in recent years.[16,17] The use of testicular sperm with ICSI has allowed many men with NOA as well as men with obstructive azoospermia to achieve fatherhood and have biological offspring. Before the advent of ICSI, there were limited options for patients with severe male factor infertility. In patients without male factor infertility, the live birth rate was 36.5% with ICSI compared with 39.3% with conventional in vitro fertilization (IVF) alone.[18] This 2015 study also found that the use of ICSI increased from 76.3% to 93.3% from 1996 to 2012 in cycles with male factor infertility present. Not only that, ICSI use increased in cycles without male factor infertility from 15.4% to 66.9% during the same time period.

ROUND SPERMATID INJECTION IN ANIMAL MODELS

In the 1990s, there were several animal studies that reported successful births and healthy offspring via ROSI. Kimura and Yanagimachi[19] in

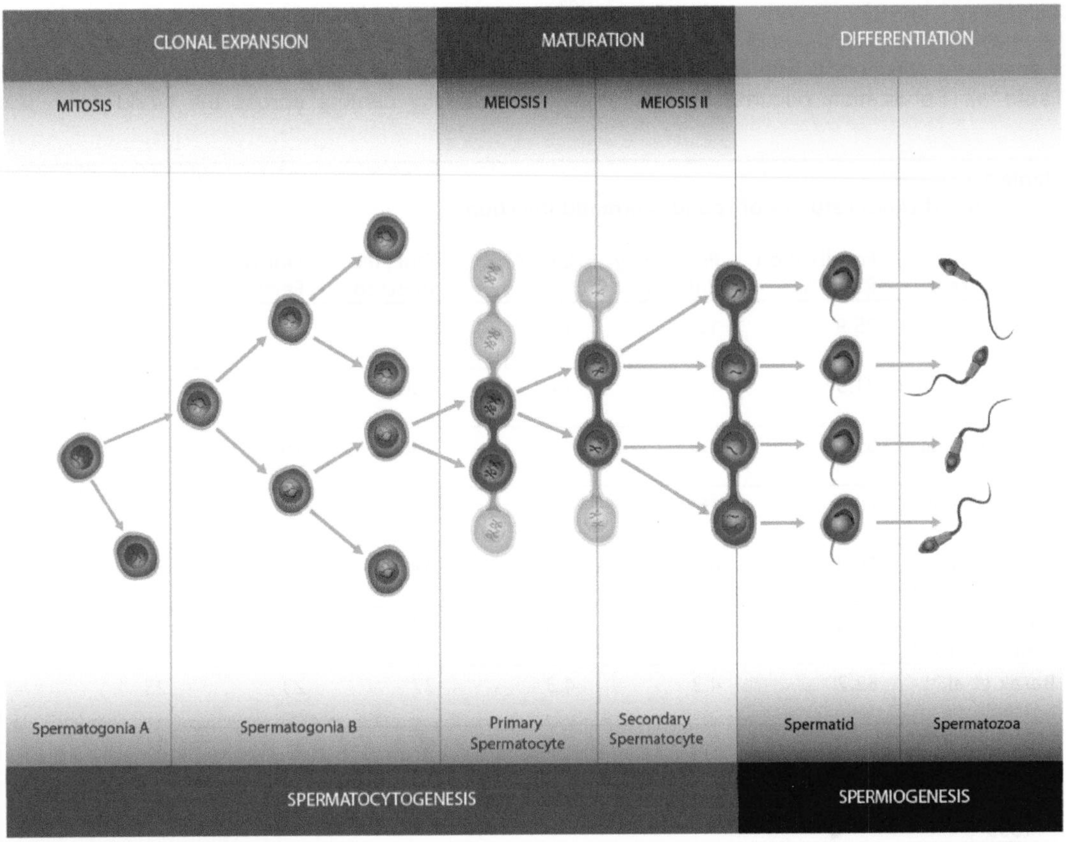

Fig. 2. Timeline of spermatogenesis.

1995 reported a fertilization rate of 77% and a pregnancy rate of 28.2% with healthy offspring in mice. They found that in the mouse, gamete imprinting happened before spermiogenesis. However, oocyte activation could not be triggered by spermatids, so this was done by electric current. Oocyte activation requires a soluble sperm factor, which is thought to be contained in spermatozoa's cytoplasm; it enables oocytes to develop a characteristic series of calcium spikes that round spermatids seem to lack, but it was found that round spermatids could be treated with a calcium ionophore.

In 2011, Ogonuki and colleagues[20] looked at fertilization of mouse oocytes using round spermatids without using artificial oocyte activation. Round spermatids in mice lack the capacity to activate an oocyte at this stage, but the investigators found when the round spermatids were frozen and thawed before microinjection, a proportion of them still developed into 2-cell embryos without artificial activation. Using frozen-thawed spermatids was thought to help with the oocyte-activating capacity in this study.

Ogonuki and colleagues[21] in 2017 studied spermatid injection in the common marmoset using immature male marmosets. The spermatids were found to acquire the ability to activate an oocyte at the late round spermatid stage. Marmoset oocytes were then microinjected with frozen-thawed late round spermatids and were able to develop to the 8-cell stage.

Despite the feasibility of this procedure, the broad adoption of ROSI has been limited because of controversy surrounding using this beyond research purposes. In addition, it must be noted that physiologic differences in the oocyte activation process between animal models and humans may exist. Therefore, certain oocyte activation protocols and fertilization techniques, which demonstrate success in animals, may not result in successful results in humans. The issue of potentially increased rates of embryonic aneuploidy and epigenetic aberrations must also be considered in humans, whereas, in animals, these issues may have a lesser role.

CLINICAL USE OF ROUND SPERMATID INJECTION

The first report of human fertilization with spermatid injection was by Vanderzwalmen and colleagues[22] in 1995. Tesarik and colleagues[23] then published a case series in 1996 of 11 cases of spermatid injection, 6 with round spermatids (**Table 1**). Fertilization occurred in 10 of 11 treatment cycles, and a pregnancy was achieved in 2 ROSI cycles, which then proceeded to live birth. However, these results were not replicated at fertility centers across the world when first

Table 1
Outcomes of clinical studies of round spermatid injection

Author, Year	Fertilization Rate, %	Pregnancy Rate, %	Live Birth Rate, %	Oocytes Injected	Oocytes Fertilized	Embryos Transferred
Tesarik et al,[23] 1996	35.9	16.7	16.7	39	14	12
Vanderzwalmen et al,[25] 1997	21.9	14.3	14.3	260	57	7
Antinori et al,[26] 1997	55.6	3.6	—	135	75	56
Antinori et al,[27] 1997	46.7	16.7	—	15	7	6
Yamanaka et al,[28] 1997	69.4	0.0	0.0	49	34	24
Kahraman et al,[40] 1998	25.6	3.1	0.0	199	51	32
Barak et al,[41] 1998	62.2	4.3	4.3	37	23	23
Bernabeu et al,[29] 1998	44.9	0.0	0.0	69	31	31
Ghazzawi et al,[30] 1999	22.0	0.0	0.0	574	126	40
Al-Hasani et al,[31] 1999	18.4	0.0	0.0	49	9	9
Gianaroli et al,[56] 1999	40.0	50.0	50.0	5	2	2
Balaban et al,[57] 2000	56.2	—	—	356	200	—
Tesarik et al,[58] 2000	53.8	—	—	26	14	—
Levran et al,[32] 2000	45.5	0.0	0.0	178	81	48
Vicdan et al,[33] 2001	28.3	0.0	0.0	69	17	5
Urman et al,[34] 2002	40.5	0.0	0.0	1021	414	16
Sousa et al,[35] 2002	15.9	0.0	0.0	126	20	9
Khalili et al,[36] 2002	21.4	0.0	0.0	42	9	6
Sousa et al,[39] 2002	34.6	—	—	26	9	—
Ulug et al,[37] 2003	41.7	0.0	0.0	36	15	10
Tanaka et al,[8] 2015	59.5	14.4	5.8	734	437	208
Tanaka et al,[9] 2018	56.8	3.6	2.2	14,324	8132	3882

Data from Refs.[8,9,23,25–37,39–41,56–58]

attempted.[24] Tesarik and colleagues stressed the importance of using the whole round spermatid, avoiding the use of just the nucleus. Vanderzwalmen and colleagues[25] published a series in 1997 of 73 azoospermic men in which 260 oocytes were injected with round spermatids. Of a total of 39 transfers, 5 pregnancies were achieved with a total of 3 term births, 1 miscarriage, and 1 ongoing pregnancy. The implantation rate was 5.5%.

Antinori and colleagues[26] published 2 studies in 1997. One study looked at 2 azoospermic men with only round spermatids. Of the thawed spermatids, 70% were found to be viable for injection. Of 15 oocytes that were injected, 7 fertilized normally. There were 6 embryos at the 4- to 6-cell stage and 1 ongoing clinical pregnancy. The second study looked at 36 patients with NOA, 19 of which only had round spermatids present.[27] Another 17 patients had elongated spermatids. Of 135 oocytes from 19 partners that were injected with round spermatids, a fertilization rate of 55.6% was found as well as a pregnancy rate of 3.6%.

In 1997, Yamanaka and colleagues[28] injected 49 mature oocytes with round spermatids from men with spermatid arrest at the round spermatid stage or primary spermatocyte stage. A total of 24 embryos were transferred, but no pregnancies were achieved. Similarly, a 0% pregnancy rate was found by Bernabeu and colleagues[29] in 1998, Ghazzawi and colleagues[30] in 1999, Al-Hasani and colleagues[31] in 1999, Levran and colleagues[32] in 2000, Vicdan and colleagues[33] in 2001, Urman and colleagues[34] in 2002, Sousa and colleagues[35] in 2002, Khalili and colleagues[36] in 2002, and Ulug and colleagues[37] in 2003, so there were clear difficulties nationwide in achieving the promising results that some centers were able to achieve with ROSI.[38]

Sousa and colleagues[35,39] in a retrospective study evaluating 159 treatment cycles in 148 azoospermic patients found injection of intact round spermatids resulted in very low rates of fertilization (17%) and no pregnancies achieved. Likewise, Levran and colleagues[32] studied the comparison of ICSI and ROSI from testicular sperm extraction samples for both and compared the results between frozen and fresh samples in a retrospective analysis of 18 infertile couples whereby the men had NOA. The fertilization and cleavage rates following ROSI with fresh versus frozen-thawed were comparable; however, the fertilization rate was 44%, which was significantly lower than ICSI (69%), and a surprisingly higher rate of cleavage arrest was found in ROSI (40%) compared with ICSI (8%). Also, no pregnancy was achieved through ROSI compared with a 50% clinical pregnancy rate by ICSI.[32] However, it is important to note that there was no method of oocyte activation being used.

In 1998, Kahraman and colleagues[40] described 20 men in whom only round spermatids were found. Of 51 oocytes fertilized, there was 1 clinical pregnancy, but unfortunately this ended in an early spontaneous abortion. Barak and colleagues[41] looked at 13 couples with male factor infertility and with 37 oocytes injected and found a 62.2% fertilization rate and a 4.3% live birth rate. Gianaroli and colleagues achieved a live birth in a single patient using frozen-thawed spermatids with 2 oocytes fertilized of 5 injected.

Similarly, in a prospective analysis, Benkhalifa and colleagues[42] assessed 14 couples who underwent ROSI and fluorescence in situ hybridization (FISH) and preimplantation genetic diagnostic. This resulted in a fertilization rate of 36% with no pregnancies achieved. Not surprisingly, only 11 out of 143 oocytes developed to have several blastomeres, and cytologic/cytogenetic abnormalities accounted for most of the blockage at oocyte, zygote, and early mitotic division stages, with only 4 biopsied embryos being normal, all of them being implanted without success.

Goswami and colleagues[43] attempted to use ROSI for treating 2 NOA patients. For the first patient, calcium chloride was used to activate the oocyte, ending in a 25% fertilization rate (2 out of 8). Using ionomycin gave a fertilization rate of 63% (8 out of 13), even though no pregnancy was achieved, and no abnormality was seen in the embryos.

Tanaka and colleagues[8] described in 2015 the birth of 14 babies from ROSI to human oocytes. All patients had undergone a microTESE, and seminiferous tubules were enzymatically dissociated and kept frozen until their use for ROSI. After thawing, through a differential interference microscope, the round spermatids were identified by their size and morphology and confirmed by FISH and karyotyping. ROSI combined with electric stimulation was used to induce oocyte activation; therefore, all oocytes were stimulated 10 minutes before ROSI. In total, 730 NOA patients that had undergone previous microTESE in other institutions participated in 163 transfer cycles. This resulted in 14 pregnancies, all of which were karyotypically normal, with average gestational age and normal birth weight. There were no developmental effects noted at 2 years. Cryopreserved and thawed spermatids yielded a better result than fresh with fertilization rates of 76.4% and 55.6%, respectively, and a pregnancy rate of 23.8% in the frozen group compared with 16.5% of the fresh sample group.[8]

Tanaka and colleagues[9] published a second study, with a total of 90 babies born by ROSI. From a total of 721 men who participated in ROSI, 90 babies were born and were followed for 2 years with repeated measures of physical and cognitive development. The fertilization rate was nearly the same as in the past study, with the frozen group performing better than the fresh sample group, 58% and 52.7%, respectively. Likewise, the pregnancy rate was higher in the frozen group with 15.8% in contrast to 5.4%. Only 3 children of the 90 had congenital malformations, all of them corrected through surgery (cleft lip and omphalocele) or spontaneously (ventricular septa). Although the fertilization and pregnancy rates are highly different between ROSI and ICSI, the 90 babies developed normally in both physical and cognitive spheres at their first 2 years after birth compared with the naturally conceived control group.

Taken as a whole, it appears that early attempts to use ROSI in humans were unsuccessful. The lack of clinical success led to a subsequent decrease in the popularity of the procedure. However, given the recent reports of higher success rates and reassuring long-term developmental outcomes within ROSI offspring, a resurgence in interest surrounding ROSI may occur in the coming years. Because laboratory techniques, embryo culture protocols, and success rates with IVF and ICSI have improved over the last decade, success rates with ROSI in the setting of a modern IVF laboratory may also improve. When evaluating the potential utility of this technique, one must consider that the laboratory environment in the late 1990s and early 2000s when ROSI was first described was quite different than it is today.

CHALLENGES AND INNOVATION

Novel methods are being tried to solve core difficulties regarding the ROSI procedure. A key difficulty many centers had was in recognizing the round spermatid under the microscope.[44] It is not easy to recognize and discriminate immature spermatogenic cells, particularly round spermatids, with complete confidence.[12,24] The identification was mainly through morphology, although round spermatids do have a similar appearance to lymphocytes.[12] It is normally a cell of 7 to 8 μm with a visible nucleus, surrounded by continuous cytoplasm; an acrosomal granule, if it appears, is a bright spot adjacent to the nucleus.[45] Hayama and colleagues[46] developed a simple flow cytometry-based method to isolate round spermatids. Similarly, microfluidics, which is a technology that uses small volumes of fluids, has begun to be used in sperm selection and testing and conceivably could be implemented in helping to identify and separate round spermatids.[47] There have also been concurrent interesting advances in using microfluidics for sperm sorting, although this is beyond the scope of this review.[48]

Another conceivable technology that could be expanded to improve the identification of round spermatids is through single-cell sequencing.[49,50] This has been used to identify markers in human spermatogonial stem cells, and the technology could be used to identify and target markers for round spermatids that could improve the rate of identification and thus likely overall success with ROSI.

There are also concerns about epigenetic abnormalities associated with improper methylation patterns owing to immature spermatozoa. There have been concerns associated with the epigenetics in assisted reproductive techniques increasing the risk of imprinting disorders adversely affecting embryonic development owing to using immature spermatids.[51] Deregulation of imprinted regions has been associated with Angelman syndrome and possibly Beckwith-Wiedemann syndrome. Kishigami and colleagues[52] found distinct methylation patterns between injections of round spermatids versus spermatozoa. Men with impaired sperm production also more often had increased aneuploidy, which may also explain the increased risk of sex chromosome abnormalities in conceptions from ICSI. The spermatid is a haploid cell with a decondensed nucleus, which is mainly composed of histone proteins, in contrast to spermatozoa, whereby the predominance is of protamines. It was hypothesized that the lower fertility rate achieved by ROSI was due to such differences in the chromatin structure affecting the consequent reprogramming of the paternal genome. Kong and colleagues[53] used a histone deacetylase inhibitor named "Scriptaid" to inhibit the typical hypermethylation observed in the spermatid-oocyte interaction, assessing for blastocyst formation and birth rate.

Precise genome editing is a promising tool for analysis of gene function; the CRISPR-Cas9 system from bacteria has been used in numerous species for modifying the genome with high sensitivity and specificity. Protocols are being developed for using this system for transplantation of the gene-modified spermatogonial stem cells-derived round spermatids for producing healthy offspring.[54] Wu and colleagues[55] used CRISPR-Cas9 to mutate an EGFP transgene or the endogenous Cryqc gene in spermatogonial stem cells after transplantation to infertile mouse testes to develop round spermatids, which were injected into mature oocytes.

SUMMARY

At this time, challenges still remain in ROSI becoming a widespread technology, and overall low success rates have limited its adoption. After initial trials in animal models, early studies of ROSI in humans had varied results and did not gain traction as a widespread procedure that could be used in azoospermic men who did not have mature spermatozoa on microTESE in large part because of difficulties many centers had in replicating the early outcomes. Recent studies have showed improvements in outcomes compared with the initial studies and on a larger scale. Broader adoption of the technology will likely need to be preceded by improvements in identification of round spermatids, although there are several possibilities that could be developed to improve the process. In addition, the possibilities are immense as to what can be done to take things beyond the current standards. There is still room for improvement in making this accessible and more successful, but feasibly allows azoospermic men to father biologic children where no sperm is seen on microTESE.

REFERENCES

1. Cocuzza M, Alvarenga C, Pagani R. The epidemiology and etiology of azoospermia. Clinics 2013; 68:15.
2. Wosnitzer MS, Goldstein M. Obstructive azoospermia. Urol Clin North Am 2014;41:83.
3. Jarow JP, Espeland MA, Lipshultz LI. Evaluation of the azoospermic patient. J Urol 1989;142:62.
4. Practice Committee of the American Society for Reproductive Medicine. Electronic address: asrm@asrm.org. Management of nonobstructive azoospermia: a committee opinion. Fertil Steril 2018; 110:1239.
5. Mehmood S, Aldaweesh S, Junejo NN, et al. Microdissection testicular sperm extraction: overall results and impact of preoperative testosterone level on sperm retrieval rate in patients with nonobstructive azoospermia. Urol Ann 2019;11:287.
6. Schlegel PN. Nonobstructive azoospermia: a revolutionary surgical approach and results. Semin Reprod Med 2009;27:165.
7. Reijo R, Alagappan RK, Page DC, et al. Severe oligozoospermia resulting from deletions of azoospermia factor gene on Y chromosome. Lancet 1996;347:1290.
8. Tanaka A, Nagayoshi M, Takemoto Y, et al. Fourteen babies born after round spermatid injection into human oocytes. Proc Natl Acad Sci U S A 2015; 112:14629.
9. Tanaka A, Suzuki K, Nagayoshi M, et al. Ninety babies born after round spermatid injection into oocytes: survey of their development from fertilization to 2 years of age. Fertil Steril 2018;110:443.
10. Neto FT, Bach PV, Najari BB, et al. Spermatogenesis in humans and its affecting factors. Semin Cell Dev Biol 2016;59:10.
11. Med ASR, Reproductive SA. Round spermatid nucleus injection (ROSNI). Fertil Steril 2008;90:S199.
12. Aslam I, Fishel S, Green S, et al. Can we justify spermatid microinjection for severe male factor infertility? Hum Reprod Update 1998;4:213.
13. Palermo G. Pregnancies after intracytoplasmic injection of single spermatozoon into an oocyte. Lancet 1992;340:17.
14. O'Neill CL, Chow S, Rosenwaks Z, et al. Development of ICSI. Reproduction 2018;156:F51.
15. Rubino P, Vigano P, Luddi A, et al. The ICSI procedure from past to future: a systematic review of the more controversial aspects. Hum Reprod Update 2016;22:194.
16. Fauser BC, Devroey P, Diedrich K, et al. Health outcomes of children born after IVF/ICSI: a review of current expert opinion and literature. Reprod Biomed Online 2014;28:162.
17. Esteves SC, Roque M, Bedoschi G, et al. Intracytoplasmic sperm injection for male infertility and consequences for offspring. Nat Rev Urol 2018;15:535.
18. Boulet SL, Mehta A, Kissin DM, et al. Trends in use of and reproductive outcomes associated with intracytoplasmic sperm injection. JAMA 2015;313:255.
19. Kimura Y, Yanagimachi R. Mouse oocytes injected with testicular spermatozoa or round spermatids can develop into normal offspring. Development 1995;121:2397.
20. Ogonuki N, Inoue K, Ogura A. Birth of normal mice following round spermatid injection without artificial oocyte activation. J Reprod Dev 2011;57:534.
21. Ogonuki N, Inoue H, Matoba S, et al. Oocyte-activating capacity of fresh and frozen-thawed spermatids in the common marmoset (Callithrix jacchus). Mol Reprod Dev 2018;85:376.
22. Vanderzwalmen P, Lejeune B, Nijs M, et al. Fertilization of an oocyte microinseminated with a spermatid in an in-vitro fertilization programme. Hum Reprod 1995;10:502.
23. Tesarik J, Rolet F, Brami C, et al. Spermatid injection into human oocytes. II. Clinical application in the treatment of infertility due to non-obstructive azoospermia. Hum Reprod 1996;11:780.
24. Silber SJ, Johnson L, Verheyen G, et al. Round spermatid injection. Fertil Steril 2000;73:897.
25. Vanderzwalmen P, Zech H, Birkenfeld A, et al. Intracytoplasmic injection of spermatids retrieved from testicular tissue: influence of testicular pathology,

type of selected spermatids and oocyte activation. Hum Reprod 1997;12:1203.
26. Antinori S, Versaci C, Dani G, et al. Successful fertilization and pregnancy after injection of frozen-thawed round spermatids into human oocytes. Hum Reprod 1997;12:554.
27. Antinori S, Versaci C, Dani G, et al. Fertilization with human testicular spermatids: four successful pregnancies. Hum Reprod 1997;12:286.
28. Yamanaka K, Sofikitis NV, Miyagawa I, et al. Ooplasmic round spermatid nuclear injection procedures as an experimental treatment for nonobstructive azoospermia. J Assist Reprod Genet 1997;14:55.
29. Bernabeu R, Cremades N, Takahashi K, et al. Successful pregnancy after spermatid injection. Hum Reprod 1898;13:1998.
30. Ghazzawi IM, Alhasani S, Taher M, et al. Reproductive capacity of round spermatids compared with mature spermatozoa in a population of azoospermic men. Hum Reprod 1999;14:736.
31. Al-Hasani S, Ludwig M, Palermo I, et al. Intracytoplasmic injection of round and elongated spermatids from azoospermic patients: results and review. Hum Reprod 1999;14(Suppl 1):97.
32. Levran D, Nahum H, Farhi J, et al. Poor outcome with round spermatid injection in azoospermic patients with maturation arrest. Fertil Steril 2000;74:443.
33. Vicdan K, Isik AZ, Delilbasi L. Development of blastocyst-stage embryos after round spermatid injection in patients with complete spermiogenesis failure. J Assist Reprod Genet 2001;18:78.
34. Urman B, Alatas C, Aksoy S, et al. Transfer at the blastocyst stage of embryos derived from testicular round spermatid injection. Hum Reprod 2002;17:741.
35. Sousa M, Cremades N, Silva J, et al. Predictive value of testicular histology in secretory azoospermic subgroups and clinical outcome after microinjection of fresh and frozen-thawed sperm and spermatids. Hum Reprod 2002;17:1800.
36. Khalili MA, Aflatoonian A, Zavos PM. Intracytoplasmic injection using spermatids and subsequent pregnancies: round versus elongated spermatids. J Assist Reprod Genet 2002;19:84.
37. Ulug U, Bener F, Akman MA, et al. Partners of men with Klinefelter syndrome can benefit from assisted reproductive technologies. Fertil Steril 2003;80:903.
38. Hanson* B, Kohn T, Pastuszak A, et al. Mp52-04 round spermatid injection into human oocytes: a systematic review and meta-analysis. J Urol 2019;201.
39. Sousa M, Cremades N, Alves C, et al. Developmental potential of human spermatogenic cells co-cultured with Sertoli cells. Hum Reprod 2002;17:161.
40. Kahraman S, Polat G, Samli M, et al. Multiple pregnancies obtained by testicular spermatid injection in combination with intracytoplasmic sperm injection. Hum Reprod 1998;13:104.
41. Barak Y, Kogosowski A, Goldman S, et al. Pregnancy and birth after transfer of embryos that developed from single-nucleated zygotes obtained by injection of round spermatids into oocytes. Fertil Steril 1998;70:67.
42. Benkhalifa M, Kahraman S, Biricik A, et al. Cytogenetic abnormalities and the failure of development after round spermatid injections. Fertil Steril 2004;81:1283.
43. Goswami G, Singh S, Devi MG. Successful fertilization and embryo development after spermatid injection: a hope for nonobstructive azoospermic patients. J Hum Reprod Sci 2015;8:175.
44. Tesarik J, Mendoza C. Spermatid injection into human oocytes. I. Laboratory techniques and special features of zygote development. Hum Reprod 1996;11:772.
45. Tesarik J, Greco E, Mendoza C. ROSI, instructions for use: 1997 update. Round spermatid injection. Hum Reprod 1998;13:519.
46. Hayama T, Yamaguchi T, Kato-Itoh M, et al. Practical selection methods for rat and mouse round spermatids without DNA staining by flow cytometric cell sorting. Mol Reprod Dev 2016;83:488.
47. Samuel R, Badamjav O, Murphy KE, et al. Microfluidics: the future of microdissection TESE? Syst Biol Reprod Med 2016;62:161.
48. Tasoglu S, Safaee H, Zhang X, et al. Exhaustion of racing sperm in nature-mimicking microfluidic channels during sorting. Small 2013;9:3374.
49. Guo J, Grow EJ, Mlcochova H, et al. The adult human testis transcriptional cell atlas. Cell Res 2018;28:1141.
50. Guo J, Grow EJ, Yi C, et al. Chromatin and single-cell RNA-seq profiling reveal dynamic signaling and metabolic transitions during human spermatogonial stem cell development. Cell Stem Cell 2017;21:533.
51. Rajender S, Avery K, Agarwal A. Epigenetics, spermatogenesis and male infertility. Mutat Res 2011;727:62.
52. Kishigami S, Van Thuan N, Hikichi T, et al. Epigenetic abnormalities of the mouse paternal zygotic genome associated with microinsemination of round spermatids. Dev Biol 2006;289:195.
53. Kong P, Yin M, Chen D, et al. Effects of the histone deacetylase inhibitor 'Scriptaid' on the developmental competence of mouse embryos generated through round spermatid injection. Hum Reprod 2017;32:76.
54. Wang Y, Ding Y, Li J. CRISPR-Cas9-mediated gene editing in mouse spermatogonial stem cells. In: Methods in molecular biology RNAi and small regulatory RNAs in stem cells. 2017. p. 293–305.

55. Wu Y, Zhou H, Fan X, et al. Correction of a genetic disease by CRISPR-Cas9-mediated gene editing in mouse spermatogonial stem cells. Cell Res 2015; 25:67.
56. Gianaroli L, Selman HA, Magli MC, et al. Birth of a healthy infant after conception with round spermatids isolated from cryopreserved testicular tissue. Fertil Steril 1999;72:539.
57. Balaban B, Urman B, Isiklar A, et al. Progression to the blastocyst stage of embryos derived from testicular round spermatids. Hum Reprod 2000;15:1377.
58. Tesarik J, Cruz-Navarro N, Moreno E, et al. Birth of healthy twins after fertilization with in vitro cultured spermatids from a patient with massive in vivo apoptosis of postmeiotic germ cells. Fertil Steril 2000;74:1044.

The Role of the Urologist in a Reproductive Endocrinology and Infertility Practice

Philip J. Cheng, MD[a,b,*], Cigdem Tanrikut, MD[c,d,1]

KEYWORDS

• Urologists • Male infertility • Reproductive medicine • Men's health
• Medical practice management • Interdisciplinary communication

KEY POINTS

- A fertility practice with a reproductive urologist helps improve adherence to male infertility guidelines and allows for better care of general male health.
- When reproductive endocrinologists and urologists work in the same practice, there is added potential for collaboration and education, which can help improve clinical care and research endeavors.
- A joint practice improves convenience and access to care by allowing couples to be evaluated concurrently and offering enhanced flexibility with scheduling surgical sperm retrievals.
- Expanding a fertility practice to include men's health can help grow a business by bringing in new revenue and increasing the patient base.

INTRODUCTION

Approximately 15% of couples struggle with infertility and roughly 7 million couples seek infertility care annually in the United States.[1,2] Male factor infertility affects about 50% of infertile couples; in one-third of cases, the male partner is solely responsible.[3] Infertile couples present to a variety of different practitioners, with gynecologists or reproductive endocrinologists (RE) often performing the initial evaluation because women more commonly initiate medical assessment for fertility concerns.

The American Society for Reproductive Medicine and the American Urologic Association have published guidelines to assist health care providers with the evaluation and management of male infertility.[3,4] These guidelines state that for all infertile couples, the male partner should have an initial screening that includes, at a minimum, a reproductive history and two semen analyses (SAs). The male partner should be referred to a male reproductive specialist for a full evaluation if the initial screening demonstrates any abnormality or if the couple has unexplained infertility.

In many instances, these guidelines are not followed. National data from the United States show that among couples who seek infertility counseling, 18% to 27% of the male partners are

[a] Reproductive Medicine Associates of New Jersey, 140 Allen Road, Basking Ridge, NJ 07920, USA; [b] Division of Urology, University of Utah School of Medicine, 50 N. Medical Drive, Salt Lake City, UT 84132, USA; [c] Shady Grove Fertility, Rockville, MD 20850, USA; [d] Department of Urology, Georgetown University School of Medicine, 3800 Reservoir Rd NW, Washington, DC 20007, USA
[1] Present address: 901 Dulaney Valley Road, Suite 100, Towson, MD 21204.
* Corresponding author.
E-mail address: philipj.cheng@gmail.com
Twitter: @philchengmd (P.J.C.); @ctanrikutmd (C.T.)

Urol Clin N Am 47 (2020) 185–191
https://doi.org/10.1016/j.ucl.2019.12.005

not evaluated.[5] According to the National Survey of Family Growth, between 2006 and 2010, only 27% of subfertile men ages 25 to 44 had received any infertility-related advice.[6] It is clear from these data that in many infertile couples, only the female partner is evaluated. Accordingly, many potentially treatable and/or reversible male factor fertility issues are left undiagnosed, which can lead to a loss of time and resources for the couple. In addition, a thorough male infertility evaluation can often reveal other underlying medical issues, such as scrotal pathologies, endocrinopathies, or genetic disorders that affect the overall health of the patient.

Most fertility centers are made up of REs and other health care practitioners whose sole focus is to assess and treat female patients. This requires them to refer couples with male factor infertility to an outside urologist for evaluation of the male partner, not all of whom are fellowship-trained in reproductive urology. To date, few fertility centers offer in-house reproductive urology services, a construct that optimizes care for the male partners and allows better coordination of care for the couple, especially if both partners require an intervention via in vitro fertilization (IVF). This article provides a brief overview of the male fertility evaluation and emphasizes the benefits of having a reproductive urologist embedded within a fertility practice.

THE MALE INFERTILITY EVALUATION

Initial Male Evaluation

The goal of the evaluation of the infertile male is to identify correctable conditions to maximize the success of conception, identify couples who may need fertility treatments or assisted reproductive technologies (ART), detect genetic causes of male infertility, and diagnose underlying medical conditions that may present as infertility. Couples should be evaluated if they have failed to conceive within 1 year of regular unprotected intercourse (or 6 months if the female partner is older than 35 year old). The physician performing the initial assessment, often a gynecologist or RE, should obtain a thorough reproductive history and two SAs.[4] The reproductive history should include the following: (1) duration of infertility and prior fertility, (2) coital frequency and timing, (3) sexual history, (4) childhood illnesses and developmental history, (5) systemic medical illnesses and prior surgeries, and (6) gonadal toxin exposure. If the initial evaluation reveals any abnormalities, the patient should be referred to a male reproductive specialist for a comprehensive evaluation.

Comprehensive Male Evaluation

A full reproductive urologic evaluation should include a thorough medical, surgical, and reproductive history; a physical examination; and at least two SAs if not done previously. The physical examination should include assessment of secondary sex characteristics and evaluation of the penis, urethral meatus, testes, epididymides, and spermatic cord to document presence/absence of the vasa deferentia or varicoceles. With regards to the SAs, reference values are based on World Health Organization 2010[7] (**Table 1**), although it is important to keep in mind that these thresholds are not the minimum values needed for conception. Based on the results of the full evaluation, other diagnostic tests or procedures may be indicated.

THE ROLE OF A UROLOGIST WITHIN A FERTILITY PRACTICE

A reproductive urologist within a fertility practice performs the comprehensive male evaluation while determining which additional testing may be necessary. Further testing may include serum endocrine evaluation (up to 45% of infertile men present with hormonal abnormalities) and imaging studies, such as scrotal or transrectal ultrasonography.[8,9] The urologist also determines whether genetic testing is warranted and provides counseling based on those results. The comprehensive evaluation may reveal other medical or urologic problems that need to be treated, such as erectile dysfunction (ED) or prostatic enlargement. Finally, the urologist determines if surgical interventions, such as varicocelectomy, testicular sperm

Table 1
World Health Organization 2010 semen analysis reference values

Semen Parameter	Lower Reference Limit
Volume (mL)	1.5
Sperm count (10^6/mL)	15
Total sperm count (10^6)	39
Total motility (%)	40
Progressive motility (%)	32
Normal morphology (%)	4
Leukocyte count (10^6/mL)	<1.0
Vitality (%)	58
pH	$\geq$7.2

Data from World Health Organization. WHO laboratory manual for the examination and processing of human semen. 5th ed. Geneva: WHO Press; 2010.

extraction, or vasectomy reversal, are necessary. In essence, the reproductive urologist creates a one-stop shop for male infertility and general men's health needs.

Adherence to Guidelines

In couples with infertility, a comprehensive male evaluation by a urologist is often not performed. One factor that explains this disparity is that the female partner tends to initiate the fertility evaluations, because studies have consistently shown that women use more health care services than men.[10,11] Another contributing factor is that, if there are sperm in the ejaculate, couples may be directed straight to IVF rather being referred to a urologist for the male evaluation. This practice pattern is likely influenced, in part, by broadening insurance coverage given that ART use has increased in states with infertility insurance mandates.[12–14]

Despite clear referral recommendations from the American Urologic Association and American Society for Reproductive Medicine, there are barriers toward implementation of these guidelines, such as a shortage of urologists with male infertility training and a lack of awareness of the guidelines. A review of 428 infertility clinics in the United States found that 22% of treatment centers did not mention male factor infertility on their Web sites and 14% did not mention any role for the male evaluation.[15] Only 23% of the Web sites mentioned referral to a urologist. Incorporating a reproductive urologist within a fertility practice allows for these guidelines to be followed routinely. If all of the REs in a particular practice can refer male patients to a urologist embedded within the practice, guideline-adherence could easily achieve 100%.

Collaboration Between Reproductive Endocrinologists and Reproductive Urologists

When REs and urologists work in the same practice, improved collaboration and education between these complementary specialties results. A survey of 336 REs performed by the Society for Reproductive Endocrinology and Infertility found that 43.5% of REs believed that their fellowship had a deficiency in male infertility training.[16] Similarly, andrology fellowships provide minimal exposure to female reproductive medicine. Some REs have argued that reproductive endocrinology and infertility (REI) fellowships should expand to include training in male physiology and infertility so that the routine male evaluation could become incorporated into their practice.[17] The opposing argument to this proposal is that even fewer appropriate male evaluations would be performed if REs deem it unnecessary to refer male partners to urologists for evaluation.[18] Furthermore, urologists are best suited and specifically trained to offer treatment of diagnoses that may arise during the course of the male infertility evaluation, including varicocele repair, orchiectomy (including testis-sparing) in the setting of incidentally discovered testicular masses, and sperm extraction. Ultimately, instead of training reproductive specialists to treat men and women, having REs and urologists work together in the same practice may provide the best outcome. Not only can this result in an improvement in care for the infertile couple, it can also enhance education and research collaboration.

Reproductive urologists in fertility centers also collaborate with their colleagues in the embryology and andrology laboratories within the practice. It is beneficial to have a close relationship with the embryology team, who can more readily team up with the urologist in the operating room during surgical sperm retrievals, and thereby improve the success of these procedures. Overall, a comprehensive center, whether colocated or virtual, affords a unique advantage for the entire fertility team to engage with and educate one other.

Sperm Retrieval

Infertile couples with azoospermia often need a female fertility specialist for ART and a male fertility specialist to perform sperm retrieval. If fresh sperm is desired for an ART cycle, the sperm retrieval procedure needs to be coordinated with the female partner's oocyte retrieval. An integrated reproductive urologist in a fertility practice can offer enhanced flexibility and ease of procedure scheduling for surgical sperm retrievals. Nassiri and colleagues[19] evaluated practice patterns for postvasectomy surgical sperm retrieval at 203 private practice fertility clinics in the United States and found that none of them had an on-site urologist. Only 40% of clinics reported performing sperm retrieval procedures in vasectomized men, with 9.4% of clinics using an on-staff RE to perform the procedures and 30.5% using a urologist who either came on-site for the sperm retrieval or performed it off-site.[19] It is evident that most private ART clinics in the United States do not have a relationship with a urologist who can perform one of the most common procedures in male infertility.

Access to Care

There are many significant barriers in access to infertility services in the United States, such as sociocultural, geographic, infrastructure, and economic barriers.[20] Mehta and colleagues[21] studied the limitations of access to care for male factor infertility and found clear geographic barriers. At the time of that study's publication in 2016, 13 states had no male fertility specialists and many ART centers did not have a reproductive urologist within a 60-minute driving distance.[21] When a reproductive urologist works at an REI practice, the problem of accessibility to a urologist is removed from the equation. Other barriers may still exist for patients, but a joint practice allows both partners to be evaluated concurrently and efficiently. This level of convenience can help improve patient satisfaction with their fertility care.

Sexual Medicine

One of the main benefits of having a urologist in a fertility clinic is that subfertile or infertile men often need to be treated for sexual dysfunction in addition to infertility. Studies have found that compared with men in fertile couples, men in infertile couples have a higher prevalence of ED and premature ejaculation.[22–24] Just being diagnosed with infertility can have a negative impact on the psychological well-being of the patient, as evidenced by higher rates of anxiety and depression.[23] An infertility diagnosis has been shown to cause an increase in stress, resulting in reduced pleasure of sexual activity and decreased sexual desire.[25,26] Treatment with phosphodiesterase-5 inhibitors, such as sildenafil, is helpful for treating ED caused by the psychological stress of infertility treatment.[27] Phosphodiesterase-5 inhibitors have been found to be fertility-safe medications that could even modestly improve semen parameters.[27,28]

Infertility and sexual dysfunction are commonly linked with hypogonadism, a problem that also should be managed by a reproductive urologist. One study showed that infertile men, especially those with nonobstructive azoospermia, had a higher risk of hypogonadism compared with fertile control subjects.[29] Treatment of the infertile male should focus on much more than just infertility given that sexual dysfunction and androgen-deficiency are often concomitant problems that persist long after helping the patient have children. A urologist that is part of the fertility care-team can easily maintain a long-term relationship with the couple and continue to manage urologic issues beyond infertility.

General Male Health

Male infertility and ED are both considered proxies for general male health. Accordingly, the role of the urologist within a fertility practice is to also assess the overall health of the patient. There is a growing body of evidence that has demonstrated an increased risk of all cancers and testicular cancer, in particular, among infertile men.[30–34] In addition to cancer, male infertility may also serve as a biomarker for other health problems, such as cardiovascular, metabolic, and autoimmune disease.[30,35–37] Other medical problems and lifestyle behaviors that have been linked to infertility include smoking, obesity, and sleep disturbance.[30,38,39] Eisenberg and colleagues[40] found that men with impaired semen parameters have an increased mortality rate in the years following an infertility evaluation.

It is important for the reproductive urologist to manage the preconception paternal health of patients not only because it will benefit the patient himself, but also for the offspring, because there is significant evidence that a man's weight and toxic chemical exposures can impact the epigenetic profile of his progeny for generations.[38] It is also critical for the urologist to identify risks of transmitting disease to offspring by offering screening and performing genetic counseling, when indicated. For instance, patients with nonobstructive azoospermia or severe oligozoospermia may have a Y chromosome microdeletion of the AZFc region, a genetic mutation that will be transmitted to all sons. REs also routinely offer carrier screening for their female patients and male partners undergoing ART to determine the risk of transmitting autosomal-recessive or X-linked genetic disorders to their offspring. When urologists and REs work directly together, genetic screening and counseling can become a more collaborative endeavor.

Business Growth

When a fertility practice employs reproductive urologists, there are many opportunities for business growth. First, expanding to male infertility and men's health creates an entirely new source of revenue for the practice. Urology is a more surgical field than REI. Accordingly, if a fertility center has its own ambulatory surgical center, an employed urologist can increase its use. Second, reproductive urologists use the andrology and embryology laboratories for serum endocrine evaluations, SA evaluations, sperm retrievals, and sperm cryopreservation, which makes the laboratories more profitable. Lastly, REs and urologists within the same group serve as a referral source for each other, which helps grow the patient base. Although the female partner of a couple more frequently initiates the fertility evaluation, reproductive urologists sometimes see male patients first, after an initial evaluation and referral by a general urologist or primary care physician (PCP). The female partner is then referred to an RE in the practice.

FUTURE DIRECTIONS

An additional benefit of having a joint RE-urology practice is the advantage of sharing the same electronic health record (EHR). Our EHR links the female patient to the male partner so that both charts are easily accessible and communication is streamlined. A future direction for fertility practices that would help improve care would be the addition of guideline-based algorithms to the EHR. For instance, for all female patients that are evaluated for infertility, there should be a male reproductive history section and order set for two SAs. When the results of this initial evaluation return, any abnormalities should flag an automatic referral to the practice's urologist within the EHR. The algorithm should automatically cue the provider to order genetic testing in oligozoospermic men, which can streamline the preliminary work-up.

There is evidence that embedding a multidisciplinary clinical care algorithm into the EHR can improve adherence to recommendations. For instance, when the 2012 US Preventive Services Task Force recommended against prostate-specific antigen screening for prostate cancer, studies showed a significant decrease in prostate-specific antigen testing, prostate biopsy, and prostate cancer incidence in the following years because of a decrease in referrals from PCPs to urologists.[41] In response to these screening recommendations, the Duke Cancer Institute created an algorithm and added it to the EHR that PCPs used, which led to an increased rate of screening among all age and race categories in their community.[42]

Many ART clinics may not be able to hire a reproductive urologist because of a lack of resources, patient volume, and access to fellowship-trained urologists. However, they can improve male infertility care by embedding guidelines and algorithms directly into the EHR, similar to the Duke Cancer Institute. Even if they are not working under the same roof at the same practice or institution, it is important for REs and reproductive urologists to maintain a close relationship so they can stay up-to-date on the ever-changing practice patterns of their counterparts.

SUMMARY

Although male factor infertility affects about 50% of infertile couples, the male partner often is not referred to a reproductive urologist for a thorough male evaluation because of poor access to male infertility specialists, practice patterns that favor going straight to IVF, and a lack of awareness of or adherence to guidelines. Fertility practices that incorporate a reproductive urologist within the practice can improve male reproductive potential, offspring health, and the general health of the male partner. Other advantages of this practice model include clinical and research advancements because of the ease of collaboration; better coordination of surgical procedures, such as sperm retrievals; and improvements in patient access and patient satisfaction. By obviating the need to refer patients to another clinic or unaffiliated practice, these constructs are able to establish a physician-patient relationship that can lay the foundation for lifelong general male health. As the fields of female and male reproduction continue to grow, more ART clinics may offer integrated reproductive urology services, allowing for optimized care of the infertile couple.

DISCLOSURE

P.J. Cheng: None. C. Tanrikut: Medical Director, Andrology Laboratory, New England Cryogenic Center, Advisory Board, Ferring Pharmaceuticals.

REFERENCES

1. Chandra A, Martinez GM, Mosher WD, et al. Fertility, family planning, and reproductive health of U.S. women: data from the 2002 National Survey of Family Growth. Vital Health Stat 23 2005;(25):1–160.
2. Thoma ME, McLain AC, Louis JF, et al. Prevalence of infertility in the United States as estimated by the current duration approach and a traditional constructed approach. Fertil Steril 2013;99(5):1324–31.e1.
3. Practice Committee of the American Society for Reproductive Medicine. Diagnostic evaluation of the infertile male: a committee opinion. Fertil Steril 2015;103(3):e18–25.
4. Jarow J, Sigman M, Kolettis P, et al. The optimal evaluation of the infertile male: AUA best practice statement. 2011. Available at: https://www.auanet.org/guidelines/azoospermic-male-best-practice-statement.
5. Eisenberg ML, Lathi RB, Baker VL, et al. Frequency of the male infertility evaluation: data from the national survey of family growth. J Urol 2013;189(3):1030–4.
6. Chandra A, Copen CE, Stephen EH. Infertility service use in the United States: data from the National Survey of Family Growth, 1982-2010. Natl Health Stat Report 2014;(73):1–21.

7. World Health Organization. WHO laboratory manual for the examination and processing of human semen. 5th edition. WHO Press; 2010.
8. Patel DP, Brant WO, Myers JB, et al. Sperm concentration is poorly associated with hypoandrogenism in infertile men. Urology 2015;85(5):1062–7.
9. Sussman EM, Chudnovsky A, Niederberger CS. Hormonal evaluation of the infertile male: has it evolved? Urol Clin North Am 2008;35(2): 147–55, vii.
10. Bertakis KD, Azari R. Patient gender differences in the prediction of medical expenditures. J Womens Health (Larchmt) 2010;19(10):1925–32.
11. Owens GM. Gender differences in health care expenditures, resource utilization, and quality of care. J Manag Care Pharm 2008;14(3 Suppl):2–6.
12. Boulet SL, Kawwass J, Session D, et al. US state-level infertility insurance mandates and health plan expenditures on infertility treatments. Matern Child Health J 2019;23(5):623–32.
13. Crawford S, Boulet SL, Jamieson DJ, et al. Assisted reproductive technology use, embryo transfer practices, and birth outcomes after infertility insurance mandates: New Jersey and Connecticut. Fertil Steril 2016;105(2):347–55.
14. Henne MB, Bundorf MK. Insurance mandates and trends in infertility treatments. Fertil Steril 2008; 89(1):66–73.
15. Leung A, Khan Z, Patil D, et al. What are infertility treatment center websites telling couples about male factor infertility? Fertil Steril 2014;102(3 Suppl):e47.
16. Barnhart KT, Nakajima ST, Puscheck E, et al. Practice patterns, satisfaction, and demographics of reproductive endocrinologists: results of the 2014 Society for Reproductive Endocrinology and Infertility Workforce Survey. Fertil Steril 2016;105(5): 1281–6.
17. Schlaff WD. Responding to change in reproductive endocrinology fellowships. Fertil Steril 2014;101(6): 1510–1.
18. Sigman M. Is it about business, education, or patient care? Fertil Steril 2014;101(6):1512–3.
19. Nassiri N, English M, Lashkari N, et al. Reproductive urologist and gynecologist involvement in postvasectomy sperm retrieval procedures at American fertility clinics. Urology 2019;133:116–20.
20. Adashi EY, Dean LA. Access to and use of infertility services in the United States: framing the challenges. Fertil Steril 2016;105(5):1113–8.
21. Mehta A, Nangia AK, Dupree JM, et al. Limitations and barriers in access to care for male factor infertility. Fertil Steril 2016;105(5):1128–37.
22. Gabr AA, Omran EF, Abdallah AA, et al. Prevalence of sexual dysfunction in infertile versus fertile couples. Eur J Obstet Gynecol Reprod Biol 2017;217: 38–43.
23. Gao J, Zhang X, Su P, et al. Relationship between sexual dysfunction and psychological burden in men with infertility: a large observational study in China. J Sex Med 2013;10(8):1935–42.
24. Kruljac M, Finnbogadottir H, Bobjer J, et al. Symptoms of sexual dysfunction among men from infertile couples: prevalence and association with testosterone deficiency. Andrology 2019;8(1): 160–5.
25. Elia J, Delfino M, Imbrogno N, et al. The impact of a diagnosis of couple subfertility on male sexual function. J Endocrinol Invest 2010;33(2):74–6.
26. Song SH, Kim DS, Yoon TK, et al. Sexual function and stress level of male partners of infertile couples during the fertile period. BJU Int 2016; 117(1):173–6.
27. Scherzer ND, Le TV, Hellstrom WJG. Sildenafil's impact on male infertility: what has changed in 20 years? Int J Impot Res 2019;31(2):71–3.
28. Tan P, Liu L, Wei S, et al. The effect of oral phosphodiesterase-5 inhibitors on sperm parameters: a meta-analysis and systematic review. Urology 2017;105:54–61.
29. Bobjer J, Bogefors K, Isaksson S, et al. High prevalence of hypogonadism and associated impaired metabolic and bone mineral status in subfertile men. Clin Endocrinol (Oxf) 2016; 85(2):189–95.
30. Choy JT, Eisenberg ML. Male infertility as a window to health. Fertil Steril 2018;110(5):810–4.
31. Eisenberg ML, Betts P, Herder D, et al. Increased risk of cancer among azoospermic men. Fertil Steril 2013;100(3):681–5.
32. Eisenberg ML, Li S, Brooks JD, et al. Increased risk of cancer in infertile men: analysis of U.S. claims data. J Urol 2015;193(5):1596–601.
33. Hanson BM, Eisenberg ML, Hotaling JM. Male infertility: a biomarker of individual and familial cancer risk. Fertil Steril 2018;109(1):6–19.
34. Hanson HA, Anderson RE, Aston KI, et al. Subfertility increases risk of testicular cancer: evidence from population-based semen samples. Fertil Steril 2016; 105(2):322–8.e1.
35. Brubaker WD, Li S, Baker LC, et al. Increased risk of autoimmune disorders in infertile men: analysis of US claims data. Andrology 2018;6(1):94–8.
36. Ferlin A, Garolla A, Ghezzi M, et al. Sperm count and hypogonadism as markers of general male health. Eur Urol Focus 2019. https://doi.org/10.1016/j.euf.2019.08.001.
37. Glazer CH, Tottenborg SS, Giwercman A, et al. Male factor infertility and risk of multiple sclerosis: a register-based cohort study. Mult Scler 2017. https://doi.org/10.1177/1352458517734069. 1352458517734069.
38. Houfflyn S, Matthys C, Soubry A. Male obesity: epigenetic origin and effects in sperm and offspring. Curr Mol Biol Rep 2017;3(4):288–96.

39. Palnitkar G, Phillips CL, Hoyos CM, et al. Linking sleep disturbance to idiopathic male infertility. Sleep Med Rev 2018;42:149–59.
40. Eisenberg ML, Li S, Behr B, et al. Semen quality, infertility and mortality in the USA. Hum Reprod 2014;29(7):1567–74.
41. Kearns JT, Holt SK, Wright JL, et al. PSA screening, prostate biopsy, and treatment of prostate cancer in the years surrounding the USPSTF recommendation against prostate cancer screening. Cancer 2018; 124(13):2733–9.
42. Aminsharifi A, Schulman A, Anderson J, et al. Primary care perspective and implementation of a multidisciplinary, institutional prostate cancer screening algorithm embedded in the electronic health record. Urol Oncol 2018;36(11):502.e1–6.

Care Delivery for Male Infertility

The Present and Future

Mary Oakley Strasser, BA[a,*], James M. Dupree, MD, MPH[a,b]

KEYWORDS

• Male infertility • Insurance coverage • Health policy • Public policy • Infertility markets

KEY POINTS

- Although infertility is considered a disease and male factor infertility contributes to almost half of infertile couples, it is frequently not covered by insurance.
- States are increasingly passing state-level mandates to include coverage for fertility evaluation and treatment, and about half of these mandates include mention of male factor infertility in some form.
- Employers are increasingly electing to include fertility coverage to improve employee wellness and satisfaction.
- Venture capital firms are investing in fertility startups and clinics, including a growing number of companies focused on male infertility products.
- Reproductive health clinics should include initial evaluation of male and female partners to deliver the most effective and cost-efficient care.

INTRODUCTION

Infertility is defined as failure to conceive a pregnancy after 12 or more months of regular, unprotected intercourse or therapeutic donor insemination.[1] According to the American Society for Reproductive Medicine (ASRM), 8% to 15% of couples are unable to conceive during this period, and male factor is solely responsible in about 20% of these couples and contributes in an additional 30% to 40% of couples with infertility.[2] Although the ASRM, The National Institute for Healthcare and Care Excellence, and Centers for Disease Control and Prevention all recommend that both partners in a couple diagnosed with infertility should receive an evaluation, one survey from the National Survey of Family Growth indicates that male partners do not receive an evaluation in 18% to 27% of cases.[2–5] Indeed, although 17% of women aged 25 to 44 years reported ever using infertility services, only 9% of men in the same age range reported ever doing so.[6]

There are numerous potential reasons for this discrepancy, including social and cultural expectations and lack of insurance coverage for evaluation and treatment of male factor infertility. Infertility has been officially classified as a disease by numerous organizations, including the World Health Organization and the American Medical Association.[7,8] However, many insurance plans in the United States do not cover diagnostic testing or treatment of infertility and instead require patients to pay out of pocket for evaluation and care, even if they have coverage for other diseases and health conditions.[9] This lack of coverage can affect patient's health as well as place significant financial burden on patients and their families.[10]

In this review, the authors assess the current state of care delivery for male infertility care in the United States. They begin by examining the scope of male infertility as well as the unique burdens it places on patients. The authors then examine the importance of insurance coverage

[a] Department of Urology, University of Michigan, 1500 E. Medical Center Drive, SPC 5330 Ann Arbor, Michigan 48109-5330, USA; [b] Department of Obstetrics and Gynecology, University of Michigan, Ann Arbor, MI, USA
* Corresponding author.
E-mail address: mostrass@med.umich.edu

Urol Clin N Am 47 (2020) 193–204
https://doi.org/10.1016/j.ucl.2019.12.006

urologic.theclinics.com

for male infertility care and current and proposed legislation relevant to male infertility. Next, they discuss the costs associated with male infertility care review increasing public awareness of male factor infertility and increasing market demand for services and coverage of infertility care broadly as well as specifically for men. Finally, this article is concluded with a discussion of potential systems-level innovations to policy, reimbursement, and practice structure to improve male infertility treatment delivery.

SCOPE OF MALE INFERTILITY AND IMPORTANCE OF MALE INFERTILITY EVALUATIONS AND TREATMENTS

Scope of Male Infertility

Male factor infertility contributes to 40% to 50% of overall infertility and affects approximately 7% of all men.[11] Despite this, 18% to 27% of infertile couples report that the male partner did not receive evaluation or treatment.[5] Given the large scope and potential impact of male infertility, it is important to consider why so few men get evaluated and the possible risks associated with this lack of care.

Importance of Male Fertility Evaluations

Evaluation of male infertility can benefit an infertile couple in 3 main ways. First, evaluation can identify and correct reversible causes of male infertility, such as varicoceles or hormone imbalances; second, it may identify irreversible conditions that may be amenable to assisted reproductive techniques and technologies, such as iatrogenic low sperm counts; third, it may identify irreversible conditions from which a male patient's sperm is not obtainable, such as certain Y chromosome microdeletions and therefore guide future reproductive decisions.

When men are not evaluated or treated for infertility, the burden of evaluation and treatment falls on the female partner. Treatments for male infertility, such as varicocelectomy, can down-stage the level of treatment and intervention necessary for couples to achieve pregnancy; as one study of 540 couples demonstrated, about 50% (271 patients) achieved a greater than 50% increase in total motile sperm count after varicocelectomy and 36.6% achieved pregnancy with a mean time to conception of 7 months, thus potentially decreasing the level of additional treatments or technology needed to bypass male factor infertility.[12]

Health Risks Associated with Male Infertility

In addition to placing the infertility burden on women, men not receiving male infertility evaluations may increase the risk that other serious medical diseases may be missed. Male infertility has been associated with a variety of significant health conditions, and evaluation and diagnostic testing can identify underlying pathology contributing to infertility and other potential health concerns. In one review of 536 male infertility evaluations, 6% of patients were found to have significant medical pathology, including 24 with cystic fibrosis mutations and other patients with karyotypic abnormalities, testis and prostate cancer, diabetes mellitus, and hypothyroidism.[13] Missing these diagnoses in male patients increases the risk that some of these genetic conditions may be passed on to offspring.

Furthermore, recent studies suggest that male infertility may be associated with increased future health risks, as summarized in **Fig. 1**. Male infertility has been associated with an increased risk of cardiovascular disease,[14] increased risk of developing germ cell testicular cancer,[15] increased risk of developing high-grade prostate cancer,[16] and overall increased mortality.[17] In one study of 2238 infertile men in Texas, patients diagnosed with azoospermia were overall 1.7 times more likely to develop cancer than the general population and 2.9 times more likely than other men evaluated for infertility.[18] Another recent retrospective review compared 76,343 men diagnosed with male factor infertility with a control group of 183,742 men who underwent vasectomy using Optum claims data from 2003 to 2016; this study found that infertile men had a higher risk of incidental hypertension, diabetes, hyperlipidemia, and heart disease when compared with those undergoing vasectomy regardless of education, socioeconomic status, race, and geographic location.[19] These studies suggest that infertility and semen quality may be a marker of overall health and that there may be a biological etiology to the relationship between fertility and future health, especially cardiometabolic health.

In addition to a direct impact on the patient's health, diagnosis of infertility has significant impact on quality of life. Couples are more likely to experience stress and marital discord; male partners in particular are more likely to report depression, erectile dysfunction, and sexual relationship problems.[20] In one study of 149 female patients undergoing treatment of infertility, global symptom scores, as measured by the Symptom Checklist-90, were equivalent to patients with cancer and in treatment of cardiac rehabilitation.[21] Indeed, multiple studies have demonstrated that psychological burden is one of the primary reasons that patients drop out of treatment of infertility.[22]

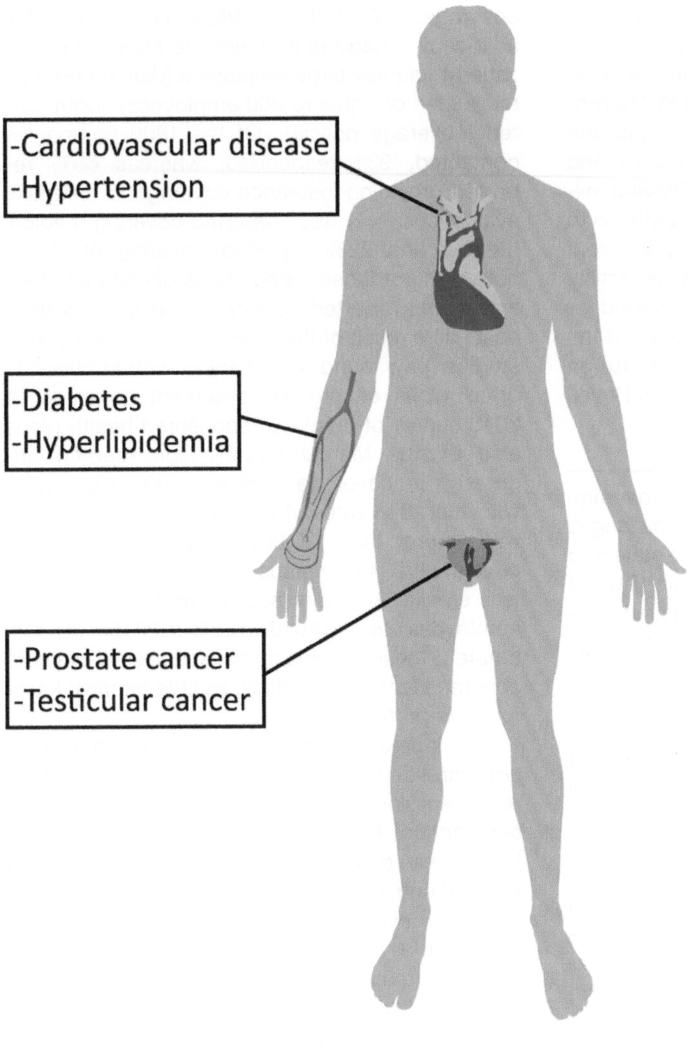

Fig. 1. Future health risks associated with male factor infertility.

INSURANCE COVERAGE FOR INFERTILITY CARE

Federal Coverage

The 2010 Patient Protection and Affordable Care Act (PPACA) remains the most recent large federal law to mandate insurance policies. Unfortunately, PPACA does not include infertility care in its list of essential health benefits and does not comment on whether insurance policies should cover infertility care, therefore leaving coverage to the discretion of private insurers and individual states.[23] Patients who are covered by federal insurance do not receive coverage for infertility evaluation or treatments. There have been 2 recent federal bills, HR 5965 and S 2960, both titled Access to Infertility Treatment and Care Act and introduced on May 24, 2018, which would have required health insurance coverage for the treatment of infertility; neither bill was passed by the House of Representatives or the Senate, respectively.

Federal legislation has also been introduced for increased infertility care, through fertility preservation, in the Department of Defense. A 2018 survey of 799 service women found that more than 30% of military women reported problems achieving pregnancy, significantly higher than the national average; the survey participants were broken into 4 categories, with the highest percentage of reported challenges (37%) in currently serving service women.[24] A similar 2014 study of 16,056 male veterans found that the prevalence of lifetime infertility was about 14%, also significantly higher than the national average.[25] As the percent of veterans involved in recent conflicts is projected to increase from 30% in 2013 to 45% in 2023, this suggests that a younger patient population with increased prevalence of infertility will have increased need for fertility treatment.[26] As a result, Senate Bill 319, the Women Veterans and Families Health Services Act of 2019, was introduced in February 2019 and "would require the DoD to provide troops the option to freeze their eggs and sperm prior to deployment to a combat zone and store the specimens up to a year after leaving military service... [and] would require the Pentagon to establish a policy for retrieving eggs or sperm from seriously injured service members whose fertility or lives are at risk as a result of a wound or illness."[27] This legislation, although unlikely at the time of writing to be passed, speaks to an increased awareness of infertility on a federal level.

State Coverage

Because the future direction of federal coverage remains unclear due to ongoing judicial challenges to the PPACA, the authors also focus on state and private insurance coverage for male infertility. At the state level, 17 legislatures have passed laws mandating the inclusion of some sort of coverage for infertility evaluations and/or treatments with various exceptions, including employer size, religious status, and type of insurance plan. These variations by state are summarized in **Table 1**. Of these 17 states, only 9 included any discussion of evaluation or treatment of male infertility.[28] Recently, Delaware enacted legislation in June 2018 that mandates insurance coverage for infertility treatments including in vitro fertilization (IVF) as well as male-specific treatments such as cryopreservation and thawing of sperm, cryopreservation of testicular tissue, intracytoplasmic sperm injections, and microsurgical sperm aspiration. It included exceptions for vasectomy reversals, religious organizations, and employers with fewer than 50 employees.[29] These exclusions include self-employed and self-insured parties, such as large health care institutions. On January 1, 2020, New Hampshire legislation will go into effect that mandates coverage for diagnosis; "medically necessary" fertility treatment; and fertility preservation for patients undergoing surgery, chemo, radiation, or other medical treatments with a risk of impaired fertility. It specifies male factor as a cause of infertility, specifically azoospermia, but does not define male factor infertility evaluation or treatments. The New Hampshire coverage does not extend to the Small Business Health Options Program (coverage option for businesses with fewer than 50 employees).

Private Coverage

In terms of private insurance coverage offered by employers, little is known about male infertility coverage. In 2006, RESOLVE, a national infertility advocacy organization, hired the Mercer Organization to survey large employers (defined here as more than or equal to 200 employees) about current coverage policies. Of the 1800 companies contacted, 931 responded; whereas 63% reported providing insurance coverage for infertility evaluations, only 39% reported covering medical therapy and 22% reported covering IVF.[30] Of note, 91% of those respondents offering infertility treatments reported no increase in their medical costs as a result of this coverage. In recent years, studies have found significant growth in offerings of all types of infertility treatment coverage. A 2018 survey of employer-sponsored health plans also by the Mercer Organization reported increases in coverage, including IVF. Compared with the 2016 rates, 15% more of organizations with more than 20,000 employees reported covering IVF (44% versus 29%). This growth trend was smaller in organizations with more than 500 employees (28% in 2018 vs 25% in 2016).[31] Unfortunately, these surveys do not specifically evaluate coverage for male infertility, so little remains know for male partners.

This increase in private coverage offered by companies potentially represents an effort to retain employees and improve overall employee satisfaction. A 2016 survey of 702 patients who had received at least one IVF treatment found that patients with employer-provided infertility insurance coverage had higher satisfaction with their employer, including higher rates of recommending their employer as a great place to work and lower likelihoods of missing work due to infertility.[32] As the average age of first birth increases (from 24.9 years in 2000 to 26.3 in 2014), there is increased discussion and surveys in the business community about the benefits of offering infertility coverage to increase employee wellness and reduce attrition.[33,34] Indeed, this is in line with justification that Delaware cited in its decision to extend its state insurance mandate to include infertility: "According to the National Conference of State Legislatures, 15 states currently have laws regarding insurance coverage for infertility diagnosis or treatment, including 2 states that border Delaware, New Jersey and Maryland. This puts the State at a significant competitive disadvantage, as many reproductive age residents intentionally change employers and leave Delaware to gain more attractive fertility care benefits."[35] Increasingly, private infertility coverage seems to be viewed as a means of increasing employee retention and satisfaction without associated increase in costs.

Table 1
Summary of male-factor infertility coverage in states with laws related to infertility coverage

State	Male Factor Evaluation and Treatment Coverage Included in Law	Restrictions	Law/Code	Year(s) Enacted
AR	None	-	Ark. State. Ann. § 23-85-137, § 23-86-118	1987, 2011
CA	Diagnosis and treatment (medication and surgery) of conditions causing infertility must be offered to employers	-	Cal. Health & Safety Code §1374.55, Cal. Insurance Code §10119.6	1989
CT	Diagnosis and treatment of individuals unable to "produce conception"	-	Conn. Gen. Stat. §38a-509, §38a-536	1989, 2005
DE	Cryopreservation of sperm and testicular tissue, storage of sperm, surgery including microsurgical sperm aspiration	Correction of elective sterilization, experimental procedures[a], religious organizations	Delaware Insurance Code Title 18, § 3342, § 3556	2018
HI	None	-	Hawaii Rev. Stat. §431:10A-116.5, §432.1-604	1989, 2003
IL	None	-	Ill. Rev. Stat. ch. 215, §5/356m	1991, 1996
LA	None	-	La. Rev. Stat. Ann. §22:1036	2001
MD	None	-	Md. Insurance Code Ann. §15-810, Md. Health General Code Ann. §19-701	2000
MA	Diagnosis and treatment of infertility, including sperm procurement, processing, and banking	Correction of elective sterilization; experimental procedures[a]	Mass. Gen. Laws Ann. Ch. 175, §47H, ch. 176A, §8K, ch. 176B, §4J, ch. 176G, §4; 211 Code of Massachusetts Regulations 37.00	1987, 2010
MT	Undefined "infertility services" as a basic health care service	Only mandated for Health Maintenance Organizations (HMOs)	Mont. Code Ann. §33-22-1521, §33-31-102 [2] (v), et seq.	1987
NH	"Medically necessary fertility treatment," procurement and cryopreservation of sperm	Correction of elective sterilization, experimental procedures[a], small businesses	2020 NH RSA CHAPTER 417-G	2020

(*continued on next page*)

Table 1
(continued)

State	Male Factor Evaluation and Treatment Coverage Included in Law	Restrictions	Law/Code	Year(s) Enacted
NJ	Diagnosis and treatment of infertility	Correction of elective sterilization; cryopreservation; experimental procedures[a]	N.J. Stat. Ann. §17:48A-7w, §17:48E-35.22, §17B:27-46.1x	2001
NY	Semen analysis; testis biopsy; correction of malformation, disease, or dysfunction resulting in infertility; fertility preservation medical treatments for people facing iatrogenic infertility caused by medical intervention; infertility drug coverage; prohibition of discrimination based on age, sex, sexual orientation, marital status, or gender identity	Correction of elective sterilizations; sex change procedure; cloning experimental medical or surgical procedures[a]; employers who self-insure are exempt	NY S.B. 6257 -B/A.B. 9759-B, N.Y. Insurance Law §3216 [13], §3221 [6] and §4303, FY 2020 New York State Budget	1990, 2002, 2011, 2020
OH	Diagnostic and exploratory procedures for testicular failure	Only mandated for HMOs	Ohio Rev. Code Ann §1751.01 (A) [7]	1991
RI	None	-	R.I. Gen. Laws §27-18-30, §27-19-23, §27-20-20 and §27-41-33	1989, 2007
TX	None	-	Tex. Insurance Code Ann. §1366.001 et seq.	1987, 2003
WV	Undefined "infertility services" as a basic health care service	Only mandated for HMOs	W. Va. Code §33-25A-2	1995

[a] Not otherwise defined.
Reprinted by permission from the American Society for Reproductive Medicine (Dupree JM, Dickey RM, Lipshultz LI. Inequity between male and female coverage in state infertility laws. Fertil Steril. 2016; 105(6):1519–1522.)

COST OF INFERTILITY CARE

Evaluating and treating infertility can be costly with high out-of-pocket expenses because infertility evaluation and treatments are rarely covered by insurance. Discussion and analysis of this financial burden frequently focuses on treatments for female patients; in particular, the high costs associated with IVF treatments are well documented in both academic literature and broader news coverage. In a 2014 assessment of 332 couples receiving infertility care at the University of California-San Francisco, 178 underwent IVF and reported average out-of-pocket costs of $19,234. Intrauterine insemination (IUI) out-of-pocket costs in this study were $2,623, and even patients who used only ovulation induction medications reported out-of-pocket expenses of $912.[36] These estimates are similar to those reported by the Society for Assisted Reproductive Technology, which estimates an average cost of one IVF cycle in the United States to be $10 to 15,000, and in the lay media, such as FertilityIQ, a Website and resource for couples with infertility, which reports an average cost of about $20,000 per cycle of IVF according to its proprietary survey data of more than 23,000 patients; FertilityIQ additionally reports cumulative IVF costs for multiple cycles averaged between $40,000 and $60,000.[37,38]

Male infertility evaluation and treatment is also expensive. In one survey of 572 couples with male factor infertility, 0% to 25% reported coverage of expenses related to medications, sperm extraction, or freezing sperm.[9] In a survey of 111 patients from 2016 also conducted at the University of California-San Francisco, 64% of men who pursued fertility treatments reported spending more than $15,000 dollars of out of pocket and 16% reported spending more than $50,000 dollars. In addition, 47% of survey participants reported experiencing financial strain due to infertility treatments and 46% reported that their treatment options were limited due to expenses.[10] The median US household income in 2018 was estimated to be $63,179 in 2018; therefore, these estimates represent between 24% and 79% of median yearly income, certainly a substantial financial burden.[39] Prices and success rates, especially for male infertility care, are not commonly listed on Websites of hospitals or providers, making it difficult for patients to make informed decisions regarding their care.[40]

INCREASING PUBLIC AWARENESS AND MARKET DEMAND FOR SERVICES AND COVERAGE OF INFERTILITY CARE

As discussed earlier, infertility evaluation and treatment frequently fall to the female partner in an infertile couple. However, there has been increased media reporting in recent years about male factor infertility representing an increase in public awareness. For example, the New York Times Parenting column discussed "what to know and how to cope" with male infertility, and Good Morning America wrote about male infertility as part of its 2019 infertility awareness week, including spotlighting several patient stories.[41,42]

In addition to this media focused on education about male factor infertility, there has been increased media attention on fear and anxiety surrounding male infertility. In 2017, a meta-analysis of 185 studies with 42,935 men who provided sperm samples between 1973 and 2011 in North America, Europe, Australia, and New Zealand reported a significant decline in sperm concentrations and total sperm counts; the study reported an average decline of 1.4% per year and 52.4% overall in sperm concentrations and a decline of 1.6% per year and 59.3% overall in total sperm counts.[43] Following the publication of this study, multiple outlets such as GQ, Newsweek, Time, and CNN reported on the results with language including "male fertility death spiral," "sperm panic," "infertility crisis," and "men are doomed;" the outlets hypothesized contributing factors to the decline ranging from stress and obesity to climate change, electromagnetic fields, and global plastics production. Although difficult to correlate, there were spikes in Google searches related to "sperm count" around the time of this study publication and publicization, as demonstrated in the data from Google Trends in **Fig. 2**.

Broadly, it seems that there is increasing public awareness and concern about male factor infertility.

Meeting Increasing Market Demand for Infertility Care

The overall demand for infertility technologies, treatments, and services are projected to grow considerably in the upcoming years. Citing increasing infertility rates and growing social acceptance of assisted reproductive technologies, various reports project growth in all areas of infertility markets. For example, the infertility drugs market in the United States, valued at 795 million dollars in 2017, is projected to grow to 922.5 million in 2022 with a 3.0% compound annual growth rate (CAGR).[44] The global IVF services market was valued at 12.5 billion dollars in 2018 and is projected to grow to 25.5 billion by 2026 at a CAGR of 9.3%.[45] More broadly, the global fertility services market is projected to exceed 27 billion dollars by 2026, more than double its 2018 value of 13 billion dollars.[46] In particular, the global male infertility market is expected to grow from about 3.3 billion in 2019 to more than 5 billion dollars by 2026 at a CAGR of 5.3%. These market reports reflect increasing demand for fertility services and technologies in the United States and the rest of the world. Growth rates are particularly high in Asia-Pacific markets, which one report attributes in part to growing fertility tourism of patients who cannot afford treatment in their home countries.[47] The bulk of revenue predicted by the market projections for male infertility arise from increasing demand for assisted reproductive technologies and varicocele surgeries, although testing and medications also make up significant portions.[48]

Capitalizing on this projected increase in consumer demand and market value, a variety of new startups are developing new technologies and services and targeting men concerned about fertility. Some companies are focusing on sperm storage. Dadi, which raised a 5-million-dollar

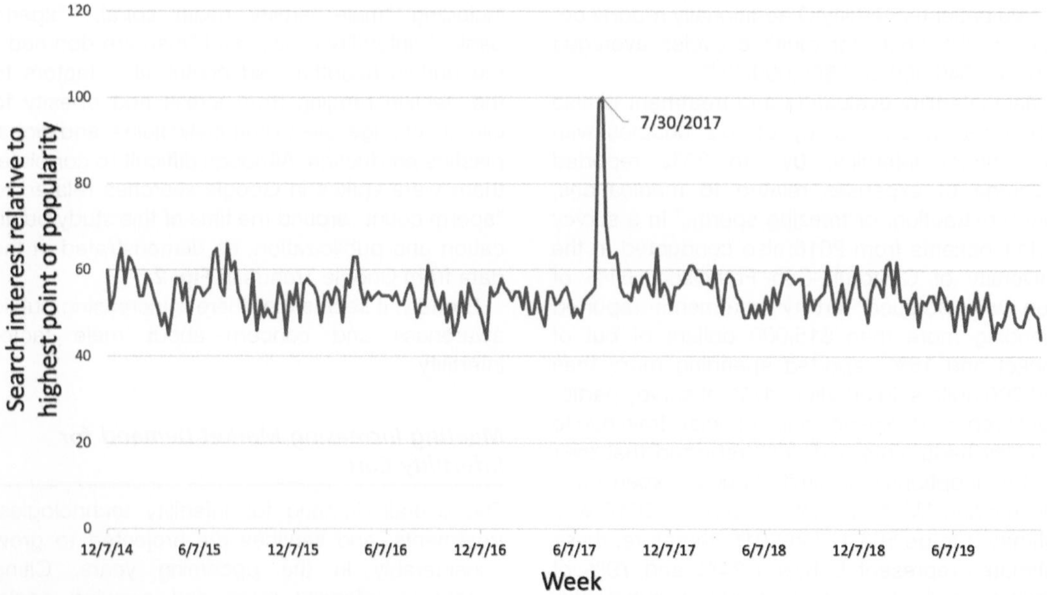

Fig. 2. Spike in Google searches for "sperm count" in July 2017, the same month of the publication of Levine and colleagues' study.

seed extension in 2019, is trying to capitalize on anxiety about declining sperm counts with advertising that urges users to "stop the clock." Legacy, on the other hand, markets itself as the "Swiss bank for sperm freezing" and raised 1.5 million dollars in a recent fundraising round led by Bain Capital. A handful of companies are developing devices that seek to improve fertility, such as Coolmen, a wearable that attaches to the testicles to keep them cool and increases sperm production (for best results they suggest wearing the device 8 hours per day). Several businesses are trying to directly address the high costs of infertility evaluation and treatment. For example, Future Family pays the upfront costs of a patient's care and converts these to a monthly payment plan for the consumer, and Carrot Fertility offers customizable fertility benefit packages to midsized companies seeking to offer this coverage to their employees.

Finally, several of these companies focus on home diagnostic devices for men. For example, the Trak Volume Cup, which retails for about 200 dollars, is a Food and Drug Administration–approved centrifugal device that allows men to measure semen volume and sperm count. The YO home sperm test, which retails for about 70 dollars, includes a microscope device that attaches to a smartphone to assess sperm count and motility. SpermCheck Fertility testing, which retails for about 25 dollars, is reminiscent of a pregnancy test with colored lines on a plastic collection device that tell the user if he has normal or low sperm count. All the devices advertise high clinical accuracies, which have been validated based on manufacturer-funded studies and published in peer-reviewed journals.[49–51] The proliferation and popularization of these types of diagnostic devices may increase the volume of patients seeking evaluation and treatment from a reproductive health specialist following at-home testing.

Potential Cost Savings Accrued from Treating Male Factor Infertility

With the media and startups helping to generate increased public interest in male factor infertility and demand for services, insurance companies may consider the potential cost-saving benefits of covering male evaluation and treatment. Varicocelectomy, for example, has consistently been demonstrated to be a more cost-effective treatment of infertility than pursuing empirical IVF or other assisted reproductive technologies. A study of the effectiveness and direct costs compared patients in 4 treatment modalities (observation, varicocelectomy, IUI, and IVF); this study demonstrated that the probability of live birth delivery following varicocelectomy was 72% versus 61% for IVF and that the average cost of delivery was \$32,171 (\$46,020 when adjusted for inflation since publication).[52] These estimates did not include indirect costs, which likely increase the total cost of the IUI and IVF routes. In another study, the total indirect and direct cost per delivery after varicocelectomy was estimated to be $26,268 compared with $89,091 per delivery with intracytoplasmic sperm injection ($42,118 and $142,849, respectively when adjusted for inflation).[53]

Patients most likely to benefit from varicocelectomy in terms of pregnancy outcomes are those with oligospermia or asthenospermia, not those with azoospermia, highlighting the importance of medical evaluation with a reproductive specialist, not just direct-to-consumer testing.[54] However, even patients with azoospermia or severe oligospermia may benefit from surgical intervention. A recent study of 17 men with total sperm counts less than 2 million who underwent varicocele repair demonstrated a mean postoperative sperm concentration of 5.4 million with 1 spontaneous pregnancy and 2 successful pregnancies with IUI (total estimated cost per pregnancy $35,924).[55] Overall, advocates for better insurance coverage for male infertility treatments may be able to leverage increasing market demand and potential patient volume with insurance providers by demonstrating cost savings of male factor evaluation and treatment.

FUTURE INNOVATIONS IN FERTILITY CLINIC ORGANIZATIONS AND CLINICAL PRACTICE STRUCTURES

With significant growth in patient awareness, social acceptance, and financial investments in direct-to-consumer male infertility startups, what might the future of male reproductive health care delivery look like? In the Glazer survey of 572 couples with male factor infertility, 71.5% were referred to a male fertility specialist, most of whom were referred by the gynecologist of their female partners.[9] This reflects the fact that the typical fertility evaluation pathway frequently still begins with the female partner visiting an obstetrics and gynecology provider, which can create tensions when different providers,and practices are taking care of the male and female partners in an infertile couple, as well as generate redundant visit costs and potentially unnecessary interventions for the patients.

Integrated reproductive health practice systems in which urology and andrology are part of larger reproductive health practices with obstetrics, gynecology, and reproductive endocrinologists represent a potentially more efficient experience for patients and likely a cost reduction for the system through economies of scale and aligned practice incentives. Ideally, a couple would present to an integrated reproductive health practice as one infertile couple and receive appropriate evaluation and testing rather than pursuing 2 separate pathways. This type of problem-based practice structure, as opposed to individual specialty clinics, allows patients to receive multidisciplinary care in one setting and facilitates communication between providers. Integrated reproductive practices are possible not only in private practice but also in larger academic health systems; the University of Utah (https://healthcare.utah.edu/fertility/) and the University of Michigan (https://medicine.umich.edu/dept/center-reproductive-medicine), for example, have Centers for Reproductive Medicine with multiple urology providers working alongside obstetrics and gynecology providers to offer tailored counseling and treatment plans to patients. In addition, some male infertility procedures may be safely performed in office-based andrology practices with local anesthesia, further adding to the value of integrated clinics. One study demonstrated an 89% cost reduction in testicular and microepididymal sperm aspiration when performed in clinic instead of the operating room and a 62% cost reduction for vasectomy reversals with similar outcomes, representing significant potential savings to the system and the patient.[56]

In addition to investment in male and female infertility startups, there has been significant private equity interest in fertility clinics. In the past, as with much of health care delivery, fertility clinics were usually stand-alone, small regional practices. In 2014, the largest conglomerate of fertility clinics, IntegraMed, only accounted for 7.7% of national market share, and 73% of the other 452 clinics had less than 0.24% market share each, reflecting the fact that most were relatively small practices.[57] Venture capital investors seek to integrate clinics into national groups with standardized best practices, newer technologies, and more flexible payment plans for patients. These are relatively recent developments; for example, in 2016 Lee Equity Partners invested 200 million dollars in an Atlanta fertility clinic and donor egg bank to create Prelude Fertility.[58] Multiple horizontal mergers with larger clinics and new locations, including a 2019 partnership with Inception Fertility in San Francisco, have made Prelude one of the fastest-growing networks of fertility clinics and the largest provider of comprehensive fertility services in the United States, already surpassing the 2014 market volume of IntegraMed.[59]

Unfortunately, based on these authors' pursual of these clinics' Websites and advertisements, the clinics seem to focus on attracting female patients. For example, the imagery on Prelude Fertility's homepage seems to exclude men; there are photos of babies and women, but the only men pictured are a gay male couple and pregnant woman with her male partner's head excluded from the frame. One Website for Colorado Center for Reproductive Medicine, which has expanded to 11 locations across the United States and Canada, includes patient education about male factor infertility but does not mention lower-cost treatment options for men such as medication or varicocelectomy. Overall, investment and expansion of fertility clinic networks in the United States do not seem to be focusing on male factor infertility evaluation or treatment in their plans for business or patients.

This investment in fertility clinic expansion means more options for patients to pursue reproductive health care; however, there are also potential drawbacks to such large-scale clinic development. Although updating technologies and merging existing clinics into national groups may help standardize care and achieve economies of scale for patients, having fertility clinics funded by venture capital could change the leadership dynamics in the clinics. Physicians may be concerned about a focus on profit returns often expected by venture capital investments. In addition, horizontal mergers between health care systems or providers are usually marketed as a means of achieving cost reduction by increasing efficiency through economies of scope and scale. However, recent studies have raised concerns that such mergers and acquisitions frequently actually result in higher costs and decreased quality.[60,61]

FUTURE DIRECTIONS AND SUMMARY

In the authors' opinion, the ideal reproductive health practice structure should include initial multidisciplinary evaluation of a couple as a single infertile "patient" with appropriate evaluation pathways simultaneously pursued for both partners. To destigmatize the male fertility evaluation process, practices could consider partnering with device companies that offer initial home testing kits to decrease the awkwardness for some patients of providing semen samples in clinic. Many reproductive-aged patients will also have higher expectations for the clinical and administrative experience, for example, online scheduling and digital communication through patient portals. Financial counseling should be offered as part of the clinic services to patients trying to navigate varied insurance coverage. Unfortunately, bundled payment options seem unlikely due to the complicated nature of fertility treatment and pregnancy outcomes; however, personalized payment plans should be considered and price estimates, including estimates for procedures, medications, and office appointments, should ideally be readily available and easily searchable.

As states increasingly mandate coverage for fertility care, more private companies elect to offer coverage as a means of promoting employee wellness, more people choose to pursue families later in life, better technology becomes available, and more patients are likely to seek evaluation and care for male factor infertility. Male reproductive health specialists should take an active role in organizing and delivering appropriate and cost-efficient fertility care.

DISCLOSURE

None (M.O. Strasser). The author receive grant funding from Blue Cross Blue Shield of Michigan for quality improvement activities (J.M. Dupree).

REFERENCES

1. Practice Committee of American Society for Reproductive Medicine. Definitions of infertility and recurrent pregnancy loss: a committee opinion. FertilSteril 2013. https://doi.org/10.1016/j.fertnstert.2012.09.023.
2. Pfeifer S, Butts S, Dumesic D, et al. Diagnostic evaluation of the infertile male: a committee opinion. FertilSteril 2015. https://doi.org/10.1016/j.fertnstert.2014.12.103.
3. National Institute for Health and Care Excellence. Fertility Problems: Assessment and Treatment. Investigation of Fertility Problems and Management Strategies. (NICE clinical guideline 156). London, United Kingdom: National Institute for Health and Care Excellence; 2013. Available at: https://www.nice.org.uk/guidance/cg156/chapter/Recommendations#investigation-of-fertility-problems-and-management-strategies. Accessed November 25, 2019.
4. CDC: reproductive health: infertility FAQ. Available at: https://www.cdc.gov/reproductivehealth/infertility/index.htm. Accessed November 25, 2019.
5. Eisenberg ML, Lathi RB, Baker VL, et al. Frequency of the male infertility evaluation: Data from the national survey of family growth. J Urol 2013. https://doi.org/10.1016/j.juro.2012.08.239.
6. Chandra A, Copen CE, Stephen EH. Infertility service use in the United States: data from the national survey of family growth, 1982-2010. NatlHealth Stat Report 2014;(73):1–21.
7. Zegers-Hochschild F, Adamson GD, de Mouzon J, et al. International Committee for Monitoring Assisted Reproductive Technology (ICMART) and the World Health Organization (WHO) revised glossary

of ART terminology, 2009. FertilSteril 2009. https://doi.org/10.1016/j.fertnstert.2009.09.009.
8. Berg S. AMA backs global health experts in calling infertility a disease. AMA: Public Health. Available at: https://www.ama-assn.org/delivering-care/public-health/ama-backs-global-health-experts-calling-infertility-disease. Accessed November 25, 2019.
9. Glazer C, Anderson-Bialis J, Anderson-Bialis D, et al. PD29-09 evaluation, treatment, and insurance coverage for infertile couples with male factor infertility in the US. J Urol 2019. https://doi.org/10.1097/01.ju.0000556129.05868.6e.
10. Elliott PA, Hoffman J, Abad-Santos M, et al. Out-of-pocket costs for men undergoing infertility care and associated financial strain. UrolPract 2016. https://doi.org/10.1016/j.urpr.2015.07.010.
11. Kumar N, Singh A. Trends of male factor infertility, an important cause of infertility: a review of literature. J Hum Reprod Sci 2015. https://doi.org/10.4103/0974-1208.170370.
12. Cayan S, Erdemir F, Ozbey I, et al. Can varicocelectomy significantly change the way couples use assisted reproductive technologies? J Urol 2002;167(4):1749–52.
13. Kolettis PN, Sabanegh ES. Significant medical pathology discovered during a male infertility evaluation. J Urol 2001. https://doi.org/10.1016/S0022-5347(05)66104-6.
14. Eisenberg ML, Park Y, Hollenbeck AR, et al. Fatherhood and the risk of cardiovascular mortality in the NIH-AARP diet and health study. Hum Reprod 2011. https://doi.org/10.1093/humrep/der305.
15. Walsh TJ, Croughan MS, Schembri M, et al. Increased risk of testicular germ cell cancer among infertile men. Arch Intern Med 2009. https://doi.org/10.1001/archinternmed.2008.562.
16. Walsh TJ, Schembri M, Turek PJ, et al. Increased risk of high-grade prostate cancer among infertile men. Cancer 2010. https://doi.org/10.1002/cncr.25075.
17. Jensen TK, Jacobsen R, Christensen K, et al. Good semen quality and life expectancy: a cohort study of 43,277 men. Am J Epidemiol 2009. https://doi.org/10.1093/aje/kwp168.
18. Eisenberg ML, Betts P, Herder D, et al. Increased risk of cancer among azoospermic men. FertilSteril 2013. https://doi.org/10.1016/j.fertnstert.2013.05.022.
19. Eisenberg M, Kasman AM, Li S. PD29-08 male infertility and future health: does the association vary by sociodemographic factors? J Urol 2019. https://doi.org/10.1097/01.ju.0000556128.98244.7b.
20. Shindel AW, Nelson CJ, Naughton CK, et al. Sexual function and quality of life in the male partner of infertile couples: prevalence and correlates of dysfunction. J Urol 2008. https://doi.org/10.1016/j.juro.2007.10.069.
21. Domar AD, Zuttermeister PC, Friedman R. The psychological impact of infertility: a comparison with patients with other medical conditions. J PsychosomObstetGynaecol 1993;14(Suppl):45–52.
22. Rich CW, Domar AD. Addressing the emotional barriers to access to reproductive care. FertilSteril 2016. https://doi.org/10.1016/j.fertnstert.2016.02.017.
23. Patient Protection and Affordable Care Act. (2010). Compilation of Patient Protection and Affordable Care Act. Available at: http://housedocs.house.gov/energycommerce/ppacacon.pdf
24. Haring E, Kirby E, Perkins L, et al. Access to reproductive health care: the experiences of military women. 2018. Available at: https://www.servicewomen.org/wp-content/uploads/2018/12/2018ReproReport_SWAN-2.pdf. Accessed November 25, 2019.
25. Katon J, Cypel Y, Raza M, et al. Self-reported infertility among male and female veterans serving during operation enduring freedom/operation Iraqi freedom. J Women'sHealth (Larchmt) 2014. https://doi.org/10.1089/jwh.2013.4468.
26. Fenstermaker M, Paknikar S, Rambhatla A, et al. The state of men's health services in the veterans health administration. CurrUrol Rep 2017. https://doi.org/10.1007/s11934-017-0733-4.
27. Women Veterans and Families Health Services Act of 2019. S.319, 115th Cong. (2019). Available at: https://www.congress.gov/bill/116th-congress/senate-bill/319.
28. Dupree JM, Dickey RM, Lipshultz LI. Inequity between male and female coverage in state infertility laws. FertilSteril 2016. https://doi.org/10.1016/j.fertnstert.2016.02.025.
29. Title 18: Insurance Code, Delaware, §3342, 3556. (2018).Available at: (https://delcode.delaware.gov/title18/).
30. Mercer Health and Benefits. Employer experience with, and attitudes toward, coverage of infertility treatment. Mercer Health and Benefits. 2006. Available online: http://familybuilding.resolve.org/site/DocServer/Mercer-Resolve_Final_report.pdf. Accessed November 26 2019.
31. Umland B, Bernstein D. The needle starts to move on reproductive health benefits. Available at: https://www.mercer.us/our-thinking/healthcare/the-needle-starts-to-move-on-reproductive-health-benefits.html. Accessed November 25, 2019.
32. Impact of infertility insurance benefits on employee/employer relationship. Available at: https://resolve.org/wp-content/uploads/2017/10/Infertility-Insurance-Infographic-Oct17.pdf. Accessed November 25, 2019.
33. Mathews TJ, Hamilton BE. Mean age of mothers is on the rise: United States, 2000-2014. NCHS Data Brief 2016;(232):1–8.
34. Kholl A. Why your company should offer fertility benefits. Forbes; 2019. Available at: https://www.forbes.com/sites/alankohll/2019/04/10/why-your-company-

should-offer-fertility-benefits/#f50976876995. Accessed November 26, 2019.
35. Delaware general assembly: senate Bill 139 original synopsis. Available at: https://legis.delaware.gov/BillDetail/26219. Accessed November 25, 2019.
36. Wu AK, Odisho AY, Washington SL, et al. Out-of-pocket fertility patient expense: Data from a multicenter prospective infertility cohort. J Urol 2014. https://doi.org/10.1016/j.juro.2013.08.083.
37. What is the cost of IVF? Society for assisted reproductive technology. Available at: https://www.sart.org/patients/frequently-asked-questions/. Accessed November 26, 2019.
38. Costs of IVF: Is IVF good value? FertilityIQ. Available at: https://www.fertilityiq.com/ivf-in-vitro-fertilization/costs-of-ivf#is-ivf-good-value. Accessed November 26, 2019.
39. Semega J, Kollar M, Creamer J, et al. Income and poverty in the United States 2018.
40. Seaman JA, Dupree JM, Deibert CM. MP46-20 finding male fertility care prices online-opaque at best. J Urol 2019. https://doi.org/10.1097/01.ju.0000556312.62054.1f.
41. Levine H. Male infertility: what to know and how to cope. NYTimes 2019. Available at: https://parenting.nytimes.com/becoming-a-parent/male-infertility.
42. What to know about male infertility, from causes to treatment options. GMA 2019. Available at: https://www.goodmorningamerica.com/wellness/story/male-infertility-treatment-options-62558954.
43. Levine H, Jørgensen N, Martino-Andrade A, et al. Temporal trends in sperm count: a systematic review and meta-regression analysis. Hum ReprodUpdate 2017. https://doi.org/10.1093/humupd/dmx022.
44. Drugs for infertility: global markets to 2022. BCC Research. Wellsely, MA. April 2018.
45. Pandey S, Sumant O. IVF services market: opportunity analysis and industry forecast: Allied Market Research;Portland, Oregon 2019-2026 2019.
46. Sumant O, Joshi K. Fertility services market: global opportunity analysis and industry forecast 2019-2026. Fremont, CA: BIS Research; 2019.
47. Asia-Pacific in-vitro fertilization amrket: analysis and forecast 2019-2029. BIS Reaserch. Fremont, CA. May 2019.
48. Male infertility market size, share and trends and segment forecasts 2026. Francisco, CA: Grand View Research. San; 2019.
49. Fredriksen LL, Epperson J, Hong K, et al. Design and validation of the trak® volume cup - a dual purpose semen collection and volume measurement device for diagnosing hypospermia. FertilSteril 2018. https://doi.org/10.1016/j.fertnstert.2018.07.777.
50. Agarwal A, PannerSelvam MK, Sharma R, et al. Home sperm testing device versus laboratory sperm quality analyzer: comparison of motile sperm concentration. FertilSteril 2018. https://doi.org/10.1016/j.fertnstert.2018.08.049.
51. Niederberger C. Spermcheck fertility, an immunodiagnostic home test that detects normozoospermia and severe oligozoospermia. J Urol 2010. https://doi.org/10.1016/j.juro.2010.07.044.
52. Penson DF, Paltiel AD, Krumholz HM, et al. The cost-effectiveness of treatment for varicocele related infertility. J Urol 2002. https://doi.org/10.1016/S0022-5347(05)64175-4.
53. Schlegel PN. Is assisted reproduction the optimal treatment for varicocele- associated male infertility? A cost-effectiveness analysis. Urology 1997. https://doi.org/10.1016/S0090-4295(96)00379-2.
54. Chiles KA, Schlegel PN. Cost-effectiveness of varicocele surgery in the era of assisted reproductive technology. Asian J Androl 2016. https://doi.org/10.4103/1008-682X.172644.
55. Dubin JM, Greer AB, Kohn TP, et al. Men with severe oligospermia appear to benefit from varicocele repair: a cost-effectiveness analysis of assisted reproductive technology. Urology 2018. https://doi.org/10.1016/j.urology.2017.10.010.
56. Alom M, Ziegelmann M, Savage J, et al. Office-based andrology and male infertility procedures-a costeffective alternative. TranslAndrol Urol 2017. https://doi.org/10.21037/tau.2017.07.34.
57. Fertility clinics: Q1. 2017. Available at: http://capstoneheadwaters.com/sites/default/files/Capstone Fertility Clinics Report Q1 2017.pdf#page=4.
58. Robbins R. Investors see big money in infertility. And they're transforming the industry. Stat News 2017. Available at: https://www.statnews.com/2017/12/04/infertility-industry-investment/.
59. Prelude fertility and inception establish the largest provider of comprehensive fertility services in the U.S. Business Wire; 2019. Available at: https://www.businesswire.com/news/home/20190328005158/en/Prelude-Fertility-Inception-Establish-Largest-Provider-Comprehensive.
60. Gale AH. Bigger but not better: hospital mergers increase costs and do not improve quality. Mo Med 2015;112(1):4–5.
61. Haas S, Gawande A, Reynolds ME. The risks to patient safety from health system expansions. JAMA 2018. https://doi.org/10.1001/jama.2018.2074.

Qualitative Research in Male Infertility

Akanksha Mehta, MD, MS

KEYWORDS

• Male infertility • Qualitative research • Health services

KEY POINTS

- Clinical and basic science research are limited in their ability to address the multifactorial challenges involved in the access and utilization of health care services for male factor infertility.
- Qualitative research produces descriptive data that the researcher must then interpret using rigorous and systematic methods of transcribing, coding, and analysis of trends and themes.
- Robustness and research integrity are just as important in qualitative research as in other forms of research and are assessed by specific criteria, including trustworthiness, credibility, applicability, and consistency.

INTRODUCTION

A diagnosis of male factor infertility has a tremendous impact on the physical and emotional health and quality of life of affected couples.[1,2] Despite this, the male partner is often overlooked in the evaluation and treatment of a couple's infertility.[3] In fact, male infertility is underrepresented as a disease, both scientifically and socially. Several barriers to access to care for male infertility have been described.[4] Foremost among these is a lack of scientific data and literature that define the scope of the male infertility problem. Health care providers and the general public, alike, have misperceptions about the prevalence, severity, and impact of male factor infertility, which compromises the quality of care for affected couples, as well as the health and reproductive outcomes stemming from treatment.

Discoveries resulting from clinical and basic science research have led to numerous advances in male reproductive health, ranging from enhanced understanding of the genetic basis of male factor infertility, to optimal management of hypogonadal men, and the development of surgical techniques for surgical sperm extraction in the setting of nonobstructive azoospermia. Indeed, such advances have made paternity possible for a substantial proportion of men previously considered infertile and tremendously improved quality of life for affected couples.

However, clinical and basic science research are limited in their ability to address the multifactorial challenges involved in the access and utilization of health care services for male factor infertility. The inability to recruit patients to participate in a randomized controlled trial comparing varicocelectomy to intrauterine insemination is a humbling reminder of the limitations of quantitative research alone.[5] Complementary approaches, such as qualitative research, mixed methods research, and/or health services research, can be helpful in identifying barriers in access to male infertility care, improving the delivery and quality of care for male factor infertility, and improve patient satisfaction.

This article explores the role of qualitative research in male infertility, including current and future applications.

Department of Urology, Emory University School of Medicine, 1365 Clifton Road, Building B, Suite 1400, Atlanta, GA 30322, USA
E-mail address: akanksha.mehta@emory.edu
Twitter: @akankshamehtamd (A.M.)

Urol Clin N Am 47 (2020) 205–210
https://doi.org/10.1016/j.ucl.2019.12.007

QUANTITATIVE VERSUS QUALITATIVE RESEARCH

Quantitative research uses numerical data to identify large-scale trends and statistical operations to determine causal and correlative relationships between variables. In contrast, qualitative research is a scientific method of observation to gather nonnumerical data in order to understand individuals' beliefs, experiences, attitudes, behavior, and interactions. Qualitative research produces descriptive data that the researcher must then interpret using rigorous and systematic methods of transcribing, coding, and analysis of trends and themes.

As such, qualitative research is ideally suited for investigating how or why a certain phenomenon occurs, rather than how often. This approach lends itself well to creating new theories using the inductive method, which can then be tested with further research. When used together, the combination of qualitative and quantitative research has the potential to more comprehensively evaluate and address a research problem, compared with either approach alone.[6]

QUALITATIVE RESEARCH METHODOLOGY

Five different qualitative research methods have been described, with Grounded Theory, Ethnography, and Phenomenology being the most common approaches (**Table 1**).[7] Data collection involves direct observations, interviews, and examination of existing documents and may be completed via individual interactions, focus groups, structured or open-ended surveys, or some combination of these techniques, depending on the study question.[8] For example, the researcher may use "small-group discussions" for investigating beliefs, attitudes, and concepts of normative behavior; "semi-structured interviews" to seek views on a focused topic or an institutional perspective; "in-depth interviews" to understand a condition, experience, or event from a personal perspective; and "analysis of texts and documents," such as government reports, media articles, Web sites or diaries, to learn about distributed or private knowledge.[9]

QUALITATIVE DATA ANALYSIS

Qualitative research yields mainly unstructured, text-based data and may include a variety of

Table 1
Qualitative research methods

Method	Description	Sample Size	Data Collection
Ethnography	Researchers immerse themselves in the study environment as "participant observers" to gain an in-depth understanding of the environment from the study participants' point of view	—	Observation and interviews
Narrative	Researchers weave together a sequence of events or experiences, as related by one or more participants, to form a cohesive story or narrative	1–2	Stories from individuals, and documents
Phenomenologic	Researchers attempt to understand participants' experience of an event or activity as well as the meaning participants ascribe to that event	5–25	Interviews, then thematic analysis
Grounded theory	Researchers explore the explanation or theory behind an event, based on the study data	20–60	Interviews, then open and axial coding
Case study	Researchers seek a detailed understanding of an event by examining multiple data sources	—	Interviews, documents, reports, observations

multimedia materials. Data analysis is the part of qualitative research that most distinctively differentiates it from quantitative research methods. It is not a technical exercise as in quantitative methods, but more of a dynamic, intuitive, and creative process of inductive reasoning, thinking, and theorizing (**Table 2**). Analyzing qualitative data predominantly involves coding or categorizing the data in order to identify significant patterns or recurrent themes or topics, which may be of interest to the researcher.[10]

JUDGING QUALITATIVE RESEARCH

Research integrity and robustness are as important in qualitative studies as in other forms of research. It is widely accepted that qualitative research should be ethical, important, and intelligibly described and use appropriate and rigorous methods.[11] That said, the criteria used to evaluate quantitative research, such as reproducibility, reliability, and validity, are not applicable when it comes to qualitative research. There are separate criteria for assessing qualitative research, which include trustworthiness, credibility, applicability, and consistency.[12,13]

Trustworthiness refers to robustness of the procedural description, that is, the purpose of the research, how it was conducted, procedural decisions, and details of data generation and management. A qualitative study is considered credible when its results are recognizable to people who share the experience and those who care for or treat them. Qualitative researchers use techniques such as reflexivity (reflection on the influence of the researcher on the research), triangulation (answering the research question in more than 1 way), and substantial descriptions of the interpretations process, including verbatim quotations from the data, to add to the credibility of the study. Applicability refers to transferability of the research findings. A study is considered to meet the criterion of applicability when its findings can fit into contexts outside of the study situation and when clinicians and researchers view the findings as meaningful and applicable in their own experiences. Importantly, although credibility refers to the internal validity of a study, applicability refers to the external validity. Last, consistency is a measure of reliability and implies that, given the same data, other research would find similar patterns and draw similar conclusions.

STRENGTHS AND LIMITATIONS

Although once viewed as philosophically incongruent with experimental research, qualitative research is now recognized for its ability to add a new dimension to research studies that cannot be obtained through measurement of variables alone. Qualitative research offers distinct advantages over quantitative research methodologies, particularly in the setting of complex questions (**Box 1**).[8] A qualitative approach also allows the opportunity to perform exploratory research in an area where there is limited or no preexisting data, in order to provide structure and preliminary data for developing a more detailed research question. However, it should also be mentioned that qualitative research is subject to some inherent limitations. First and foremost is the potential for the mere presence of the researcher to influence the subjects' responses. The researcher's ability and training in qualitative research methodologies can further affect the quality of the work. Last, qualitative data analysis and summary can be time consuming, often requiring a second analyst to ensure consistency.[8]

APPLICATIONS TO MALE INFERTILITY

The cause of male infertility is multifactorial. Utilization of services for the diagnosis and treatment

Table 2
Overview of qualitative data preparation and analysis

Step 1: Become familiar with the data	Transcribe the data, if applicable. Read and review the data several times in order to become familiar with it. Start looking for basic observations and patterns.
Step 2: Revisit research objectives	Revisit the research objective and identify the questions that can be answered through the collected data.
Step 3: Develop a framework	Identify broad ideas, concepts, behaviors, and assign labels/codes to them in order to organize them into groups. This is helpful for structuring the data.
Step 4: Identify patterns and connections	Start identifying themes, looking for the most common behaviors or responses from study participants, identifying patterns that can answer research questions, and finding areas that can be explored further.

Box 1
Strengths and limitations of qualitative research

Strengths of qualitative research

- Research questions can be examined in detail and in depth; all subtleties and complexities can be fully explored
- Interviews can be structured and guided by the researcher in real time, depending on the responses being provided by the study participants
- The research framework and direction can be revised/updated as new information emerges
- Data based on human experience can be more engaging and compelling than numerical data
- Research findings can be transferable to another setting

Limitations of qualitative research

- Research quality is dependent on the individual skill of the researcher
- Data analysis and interpretation can be time consuming
- The researcher's presence during data collection, which is unavoidable, can itself affect subjects' responses
- Results can be difficult to summarize in a visual manner

of male infertility is, similarly, dependent on several factors.[4] Qualitative research methodology is, therefore, ideally suited to try and understand how and why affected patients decide to seek care, how care delivery can be optimized, and how patient satisfaction and clinical outcomes can be improved. The following sections describe 2 examples of topics whereby qualitative approaches have been applied in male infertility and reproductive health research.

Knowledge About Male Factor Infertility

Infertility has traditionally been considered a female problem, and resources related to infertility diagnosis, counseling, and treatment have disproportionately focused on the female partner. Although men aspire to parenthood just as much as women, the literature suggests that men have poor knowledge about the factors that influence fertility.[14–17] In addition, men overestimate the chance of spontaneous and assisted conception, which is especially problematic in an era whereby the gap between ideal biological and ideal social age for having children is widening, thereby narrowing the timeframe in which parenthood can be achieved.[14]

A recent qualitative study of men's attitudes and preferences toward family formation provides some insight into this disconnect between the desire for paternity, on 1 hand, and the tendency to delay family building on the other.[18] Through a series of semistructured interviews, Sylvest and colleagues[18] found that even men who desire a nuclear family with biologically related children feel ambivalence about parenthood and feeling "ready." In their analysis, the lack of readiness was linked to men's awareness of the sacrifices and costs involved with parenthood, and their belief that they could safely delay parenthood. The men participating in the study did not, in fact, consider that they may be unable to have their own biological children.

Indeed, a diagnosis of male factor infertility can come as a surprise to many men.[19] It is well accepted that men and women experience infertility differently. The diagnosis can be a distressing experience for men, because of stigma, threats to masculinity, and the perceived need to suppress emotions.[20] Several studies have examined the online emoting of men in relation to infertility via anonymous forum posts on men-only infertility discussion boards. In general, these analyses demonstrate men's psychological needs for vocalizing the emotional burdens of infertility, personal coping strategies, and relationships with other men who are going through similar experiences.[20–22]

Male and female representation and participation in discussions about fertility and reproductive health differ greatly. Based on interviews of men and women of reproductive age, and their physicians, Grace and colleagues[23] found that although men generally wanted to improve their fertility knowledge, and be involved in family building discussions, they thought they did not have a voice on the topic because such discussions have traditionally focused on women. Health care professionals agreed that fertility was perceived as the woman's domain, but also highlighted that poor male involvement is typically observed across health care needs and is not necessarily unique to fertility and reproductive health.[23] In light of these findings, it seems the notion that men are not interested or engaged in reproductive concerns becomes somewhat of a self-fulfilling prophecy.

Taken together, these studies illustrate that knowledge about male factor infertility is lacking among men of reproductive age for several interrelated reasons. Improving gaps in knowledge is likely to require more than just dissemination of written or verbal information pertaining to male factor infertility; it will ultimately require a shift in societal perceptions of male and female factor infertility, and destigmatization of the psychological impact of a diagnosis of infertility for all affected patients.

Experience of Oncofertility and Survivorship Counseling

Qualitative research methods, such as interviews and surveys, have been frequently used to assess the fertility-associated concerns of patients with cancer, as well as their attitudes toward fertility preservation. A growing body of literature confirms that future paternity is an important concern among cancer survivors, and that failure to address reproductive concerns before undergoing cancer therapy is associated with subsequent distress and regret.[24–26]

As a complement to the existing data, a recent qualitative study demonstrates the tangible benefit of offering oncofertility care to patients with cancer. Wang and colleagues[27] conducted semistructured interviews of newly diagnosed patients with cancer of reproductive age, to explore the fertility care experiences and reproductive concerns of patients with cancer who had access to oncofertility care at the time of their cancer diagnosis. Thematic analysis identified the 5 following main themes: (i) satisfaction with oncofertility care, (ii) a need for individualized treatment and support, (iii) desire for parenthood, (iv) the fact that fertility treatment can be challenging, and (v) the fact that fertility preservation provides a safety net for the future. The investigators concluded patients who access supportive oncofertility care experience low emotional impact of threatened future infertility at the time of cancer diagnosis, and that oncofertility services can assist in lowering the emotional burden of potential infertility in survivors.[27]

MIXED METHODS RESEARCH

It is possible to combine quantitative and qualitative methods, either sequentially (first a quantitative and then a qualitative study or vice versa), where the first approach is used to facilitate the design of the second; in parallel, as different approaches to the same question; or by enriching a dominant method with a small component of an alternative method (such as qualitative interviews "nested" in a large survey). However, this combination of quantitative and qualitative research methods, termed a "mixed methods approach," must be carefully and intentionally designed, to ensure that the theory behind each method is compatible and that the methods are being used for appropriate reasons. A random combination of quantitative and qualitative data, for example, a free text field in a multiple-choice-item survey, does not constitute mixed methods research.

Qualitative and quantitative methods may be used together for corroboration (hoping for similar outcomes from both methods), elaboration (using qualitative data to explain or interpret quantitative data, or to demonstrate how the quantitative findings apply in particular cases), complementarity (where the qualitative and quantitative results differ but generate complementary insights), or contradiction (where qualitative and quantitative data lead to different conclusions).[9]

Appropriate and specific data analysis techniques must also be used in the setting of mixed methods research, rather than a random amalgam of quantitative and qualitative techniques.

SUMMARY

In summary, qualitative research methods represent a valuable tool for investigating the entirety of the experience of male infertility evaluation, diagnosis, and treatment. Qualitative research is rigorous and thorough and well adapted for studying the complex field of infertility and reproductive health. Knowledge gained from qualitative research methods can undoubtedly inform clinical practice and improve support for individuals and couples affected by male factor infertility.

DISCLOSURE

Dr. A. Mehta is supported by a Research Grant from the American Society for Reproductive Medicine.

REFERENCES

1. Smith JF, Walsh TJ, Shindel AW, et al. Sexual, marital, and social impact of a man's perceived infertility diagnosis. J Sex Med 2009;6(9):2505–15.
2. Walschaerts M, Bujan L, Parinaud J, et al. Treatment discontinuation in couples consulting for male infertility after failing to conceive. Fertil Steril 2013;99(5):1319–23.
3. Petok WD. Infertility counseling (or the lack thereof) of the forgotten male partner. Fertil Steril 2015; 104(2):260–6.
4. Mehta A, Nangia AK, Dupree JM, et al. Limitations and barriers in access to care for male factor infertility. Fertil Steril 2016;105(5):1128–37.
5. Trussell JC, Christman GM, Ohl DA, et al. Recruitment challenges of a multicenter randomized controlled varicocelectomy trial. Fertil Steril 2011; 96(6):1299–305.

6. Brannen J. Mixing methods: the entry of qualitative and quantitative approaches into the research process. Int J Soc Res Methodol 2005;8(3):173–84.
7. Denzin NK, Lincoln YS. The SAGE handbook of qualitative research. 4th edition. Thousand Oaks, CA: SAGE Publications; 2011.
8. Anderson C. Presenting and evaluating qualitative research. Am J Pharm Educ 2010;74(8):141.
9. Hammarberg K, Kirkman M, de Lacey S. Qualitative research methods: when to use them and how to judge them. Hum Reprod 2016;31(3):498–501.
10. Patton MQ. Qualitative research and evaluation methods. 3rd. edition. Thousand Oaks, CA: SAGE Publications.; 2002.
11. Cohen DJ, Crabtree BF. Evaluative criteria for qualitative research in health care: controversies and recommendations. Ann Fam Med 2008;6(4):331–9.
12. Dixon-Woods M, Sutton A, Shaw R, et al. Appraising qualitative research for inclusion in systematic reviews: a quantitative and qualitative comparison of three methods. J Health Serv Res Policy 2007; 12(1):42–7.
13. Kitto SC, Chesters J, Grbich C. Quality in qualitative research. Med J Aust 2008;188(4):243–6.
14. Hammarberg K, Collins V, Holden C, et al. Men's knowledge, attitudes and behaviours relating to fertility. Hum Reprod Update 2017;23(4):458–80.
15. Daniluk JC, Koert E. Fertility awareness online: the efficacy of a fertility education website in increasing knowledge and changing fertility beliefs. Hum Reprod 2015;30(2):353–63.
16. Daniluk JC, Koert E. The other side of the fertility coin: a comparison of childless men's and women's knowledge of fertility and assisted reproductive technology. Fertil Steril 2013;99(3):839–46.
17. Daumler D, Chan P, Lo KC, et al. Men's knowledge of their own fertility: a population-based survey examining the awareness of factors that are associated with male infertility. Hum Reprod 2016; 31(12):2781–90.
18. Sylvest R, Koert E, Birch Petersen K, et al. Attitudes towards family formation among men attending fertility counselling. Reprod Biomed Soc Online 2018;6:1–9.
19. Mehta A, Hanson B, Hawkins C, et al. Qualitative analysis of male partner needs among infertile couples. J Urol 2019;201:e555.
20. Hanna E, Gough B. Emoting infertility online: a qualitative analysis of men's forum posts. Health (London) 2016;20(4):363–82.
21. Hanna E, Gough B. Searching for help online: an analysis of peer-to-peer posts on a male-only infertility forum. J Health Psychol 2018;23(7):917–28.
22. Richard J, Badillo-Amberg I, Zelkowitz P. "So much of this story could be me": men's use of support in online infertility discussion boards. Am J Mens Health 2017;11(3):663–73.
23. Grace B, Shawe J, Johnson S, et al. You did not turn up... I did not realise I was invited... understanding male attitudes towards engagement in fertility and reproductive health discussions. Hum Reprod Open 2019;2019(3):hoz014.
24. Schover LR, Brey K, Lichtin A, et al. Knowledge and experience regarding cancer, infertility, and sperm banking in younger male survivors. J Clin Oncol 2002;20(7):1880–9.
25. Saito K, Suzuki K, Iwasaki A, et al. Sperm cryopreservation before cancer chemotherapy helps in the emotional battle against cancer. Cancer 2005; 104(3):521–4.
26. Dohle GR. Male infertility in cancer patients: review of the literature. Int J Urol 2010;17(4):327–31.
27. Wang Y, Logan S, Stern K, et al. Supportive oncofertility care, psychological health and reproductive concerns: a qualitative study. Support Care Cancer 2019. https://doi.org/10.1007/s00520-019-04883-1.

Male Infertility and Somatic Health

Mujalli Mhailan Murshidi, MD, FRCS (England)[a,b,1], Jeremy T. Choy, MD[c], Michael L. Eisenberg, MD[d,*]

KEYWORDS

• Male infertility • Men's health • Somatic health

KEY POINTS

- Somatic health is associated with male infertility.
- Potential links between male infertility and health include genetic, developmental, and lifestyle factors.
- Male infertility also may be a predictor of oncologic, cardiovascular, metabolic, autoimmune diseases, hospitalization and mortality.
- Additional research is required to elucidate the mechanisms by which male infertility affects overall health.

INTRODUCTION

Humankind has been interested in reproduction for millennia, as it is the primary instinct of all organisms and it is a social, cultural, and medical issue. Infertility and surrogacy are first mentioned on a 4000-year-old Assyrian clay tablet of a marriage contract exhibited at Istanbul Archeology Museum in Turkey.[1]

Infertility is defined as the inability to conceive after 1 year of unprotected intercourse.[2] Agarwal and colleagues[3] documented that the estimated number of couples with infertility worldwide is 48.5 million and calculated rates of male infertility across the globe.

Approximately 15% of couples are affected by infertility, with male factor infertility thought to play a role in 50% of infertile couples, acting as the sole contributor in 20% to 30% of infertility cases.[4,5] There exists a growing body of literature that would suggest an association between male infertility and a host of other medical conditions, including oncologic, cardiovascular, autoimmune, and other chronic diseases, to broader outcomes such as hospitalizations and mortality. The exact nature of these associations remains unclear, although popular hypothesized etiologic mechanisms include genetic, developmental, and lifestyle-based factors. The purpose of this review was to survey the existing data of these associations, to provide a better understanding of the relationship between male infertility and overall somatic health, in addition explore some of the new ideas in the field.

GENETIC ASSOCIATIONS

Given that approximately 10% of the human genome is involved in reproduction, it is reasonable to assume that a genetic mutation affecting

[a] The University of Jordan, Amman, Jordan; [b] Department of Urology, Stanford University School of Medicine, Stanford, CA, USA; [c] Endocrinology, Department of Medicine, Stanford University School of Medicine, Stanford, CA, USA; [d] Male Reproductive Medicine and Surgery, Department of Urology, Stanford University School of Medicine, Stanford, CA, USA
[1] Mujalli Mhailan Murshidi conducted his role during sabbatical leave at Stanford University from the University of Jordan.
* Corresponding author.
E-mail address: eisenberg@stanford.edu
Twitter: @drmeisenberg (M.L.E.)

Urol Clin N Am 47 (2020) 211–217
https://doi.org/10.1016/j.ucl.2019.12.008

reproduction could also affect another organ system. For example, Klinefelter syndrome (47, XXY genotype) is a genetic cause of primary hypogonadism, which leads to male infertility in addition to the extragonadal phenotypic manifestations of the syndrome, such as an increased risk of cardiovascular disease, metabolic syndrome, insulin resistance, diabetes mellitus, and cancer.[6–8] Another classic example is a mutation in the cystic fibrosis transmembrane conductance regulator (*CFTR*) gene, which can result in congenital bilateral absence of the vas deferens or epididymal obstruction leading to male infertility, while also giving rise to a cystic fibrosis phenotype.[9]

Next, mutations in the *MLH1* gene, which give rise to Lynch syndrome, also have been identified in men with nonobstructive azoospermia (NOA).[10] *ERCC1* and *MSH2* are other genes that have been found to be involved in DNA mismatch repair,[11,12] nonobstructive azoospermia, and the development of colorectal cancers.[13,14] In addition, there is evidence that men with NOA demonstrate higher rates of defects in DNA repair mechanisms and cell cycle regulation, and higher rates of cancer have been found in azoospermic men.[15,16] Next, men with NOA also have shorter telomere lengths, which have been associated with premature aging.

Deletions involving the Y chromosome can impair spermatogenesis.[17] Y chromosome microdeletions can also involve the *SHOX* (short-stature homeobox) gene, the haploinsufficiency of which can give rise to short stature.[18] It was found recently that there is a relationship of 4 potentially functional polymorphisms associated with oxidative stress pathway genes (superoxide dismutase-SOD2 Ile58Thr and SOD2 rs4880, catalase-CAT C-262T, glutathione peroxidase 1-GPX1 Pro200Leu) and increased male infertility risk.[19]

In addition, Ben Rhouma and colleagues[20] stated that 33 genes have been identified as responsible for nonsyndromic male infertility. The evolution of techniques based on whole-genome analysis has allowed the development of more successful methods in the identification of new genes and mutations inducing an infertility phenotype. As such, new genetic links between reproductive and somatic health are likely to arise.

DEVELOPMENTAL ASSOCIATIONS

Hypothesized by David Barker,[21] the concept of fetal origins of adult disease posits that intrauterine events can impact an individual's risk of developing diseases in adult life.[22] In a similar way, the testicular dysgenesis syndrome (TDS), introduced by Skakkebaek and collegues,[23] suggests in utero exposures can alter normal genital growth and development. TDS links several male genital anomalies, including poor semen quality, hypospadias, cryptorchidism, and testicular cancer. Although the causes are unclear, environmental exposures, including chemical exposures or assisted reproductive technologies, have been suggested.[24] Indeed, children conceived through in vitro fertilization and intracytoplasmic sperm injection have been found to have higher rates of cryptorchidism and hypospadias, as well as higher rates of preterm birth and low birth weight.[25] In addition, preterm infants are at higher risk for a variety of systemic diseases, including cardiovascular disease and diabetes.[26,27] Next, studies have demonstrated that young men conceived via intracytoplasmic sperm injection have lower sperm concentrations and total sperm counts compared with boys conceived without assistance[28] On the other hand, among men undergoing infertility evaluation, there is no significant relationship between semen parameters and defect rates in live or still births, even when considering mode of conception.[29]

LIFESTYLE ASSOCIATIONS

In a similar way that many lifestyle factors are associated with the development of chronic disease, studies suggest a relationship between lifestyle factors and male infertility. Current data suggest that obesity negatively impacts male fertility. A meta-analysis of 21 studies, including those performed by Sermondade and colleagues,[30] demonstrated that as body mass index (BMI) increased, so did the odds of oligospermia and azoospermia. BMI provides another link between fertility and chronic disease, as overweight and obese men are at risk for adverse health outcomes. Obesity was associated with lower semen volume, lower sperm motility, and erectile dysfunction in infertile couples.[31] However, there is sufficient literature to support that weight reduction by diet and exercise, smoking cessation, and alcohol moderation are positive in male fertility.

Certain lifestyle habits, such as tobacco use, have negative health and reproductive effects. A meta-analysis performed by Li and colleagues[32] showed that smoking is an independent risk factor for reduced semen quality. In contrast, the association between male fertility and alcohol consumption is uncertain, as studies have suggested that moderate alcohol intake is not adversely associated with semen quality.[33] Another study found no association with the probability of conception and alcohol consumption in men.[34]

Next, there is increasing evidence that current health is associated with male fertility. Salonia and colleagues[35] demonstrated that infertile men had a significantly higher rate of comorbidities (as measured by the Charlson Comorbidity Index [CCI]) in comparison with their fertile controls. A subsequent cross-sectional study of 9387 men showed that increasing CCIs were associated with decreased semen volume, sperm concentration, sperm total count, and sperm motility. When looking at specific comorbidities, men with hypertension, cardiac disease, and peripheral vascular disease were found to have increased rates of seminal parameter abnormalities.[27] In addition, there is evidence that treatment of medical comorbidities can improve fertility. Shiraishi and Matsuyama[36] found that men who were successfully treated for various medical comorbidities (eg, hypertension, hyperlipidemia) had significant improvements in their total motile sperm counts.

Infectious etiologies may also affect somatic and reproductive health. For example, schistosomiasis, which is endemic in some developing countries, may induce infertility, due to hormonal imbalance, testicular tissue damage, and genital ductal system obstruction.[37] Human papillomavirus (HPV) may be risk factor for male infertility, as some studies have shown a higher prevalence of high-risk HPV in infertile men than fertile men.[38]

MALE INFERTILITY AND ONCOLOGIC DISEASE

Cancer and its therapy can impair male fertility.[39] However, emerging evidence suggests a link between male infertility and risk of incident malignant disease. The best-studied example is the association between infertility and testicular cancer. Many groups have explored this relationship. A Danish cohort study examined more than 30,000 men and reported that low sperm concentration, decreased sperm motility, and poorer sperm morphology were each independently associated with an increased incidence of testicular cancer.[40] In addition, a large American multicenter cohort study of more than 51,000 infertile couples in California found that diagnosed male factor infertility was associated with a nearly threefold increase in the incidence of testicular cancer.[41] Another American study used commercial insurance claims data to examine more than 75,000 infertile men and found that the group of infertile men had higher rates of all cancers, testicular cancer, as well as non-Hodgkin lymphoma.[42] Although the etiology between male infertility and testicular cancer require more study, as discussed earlier, hypothesized potential mechanisms include developmental, genetic, and environmental etiologic factors.

A link between infertility and prostate cancer is uncertain, with conflicting data in the literature. A 2010 retrospective cohort study looking at 22,562 California men who had undergone fertility testing demonstrated that men with infertility were at an increased risk for developing high-grade prostate cancer but not overall prostate cancer.[43] Conversely, a 2016 retrospective cohort study of 20,433 men who underwent semen analysis found no association between infertility and prostate cancer risk.[44] In addition, a Swedish nested case-control study of 445 patients with prostate cancer reported lower odds of developing prostate cancer in infertile men.[45]

Interestingly, there are recent data suggesting that male infertility may serve not only as a biomarker for an individual man's health, but also as a marker of oncologic risk for the affected man's family members.[46] A 2016 study revealed that first-degree relatives of the men who underwent semen analysis had a 52% increased risk of testicular cancer, as compared with the first-degree relatives of the fertile controls. In addition, first-degree and second-degree relatives of men with azoospermia were found to have an increased risk of thyroid cancer.[47] Furthermore, a subsequent retrospective cohort study of 10,511 men from Utah who had undergone semen analysis and their 63,891 siblings and 327,753 cousins revealed that oligospermia was associated with a twofold increase in risk of childhood cancer in the subfertile man's siblings, as well as a threefold risk of specifically acute lymphoblastic leukemia in the siblings, as compared with the siblings of fertile controls.[48] Although the origins of these familial associations are unclear, shared genetics or environment provide plausible mechanisms.

MALE INFERTILITY AND NONONCOLOGIC CHRONIC DISEASES

An association also has been suggested between male infertility and cardiometabolic disease. Although prevalent cardiovascular disease is associated with impaired semen quality, as a recent study found hypertensive men to have lower seminal volume, sperm count, and sperm motility compared with men without the diagnosis of hypertension,[49] the question of incident cardiovascular disease after a male infertility diagnosis is uncertain. To date, many of the studies undertaken thus far have used surrogate markers for infertility, thus limiting the interpretability of the data. For example, one study assessed fatherhood (ie, having children or not) and the risk of cardiovascular disease using data from the National Institutes of Health–AARP Diet and Health Study, and found that childless men had an increased risk of death from cardiovascular disease compared with fathers.[50] However, childlessness serves as an imperfect surrogate for infertility, given that childless men may not necessarily be infertile.

A study examining US insurance claims data demonstrated that men diagnosed with male factor infertility were at increased risk of developing ischemic heart disease relative to control groups.[51] In addition, a US study noted that men with varicoceles have a higher incidence of heart disease.[52] Although varicoceles may contribute to male infertility, the presence of a varicocele does not necessarily imply infertility.

Given that low semen quality is associated with obesity,[30] further work has suggested that lipid concentrations may negatively impact semen parameters, as higher serum levels of total cholesterol and phospholipids have been associated with poorer sperm morphology.[53] Other studies have identified an increased prevalence of infertility in men with type 2 diabetes mellitus,[54] as well as increased risk of incident diabetes among those diagnosed with male factor infertility.[51]

A Danish study of more than 24,000 infertile men demonstrated that infertile men had higher risk of both prevalent and incident multiple sclerosis.[55] Given the suspected autoimmune nature of the pathogenesis of multiple sclerosis, another study used insurance claims data to assess for a relationship between male infertility and autoimmune diseases, and found that a cohort of infertile men had a higher risk of developing incident rheumatoid arthritis, psoriasis, multiple sclerosis, Graves' disease, and autoimmune thyroiditis.[56] Although the mechanism of the proposed association between infertility and autoimmunity remains unclear, evidence suggests that androgens may modulate immunity.[57]

In addition, a Danish study of men evaluated for infertility found that decreased sperm concentration, total sperm count, and sperm motility were associated with increased rates of all-cause hospitalizations. Specifically, sperm concentrations less than 15 million/mL were clearly associated with an increased risk of being hospitalized.[58] As with earlier work, causation remains uncertain. Factors related to health or lifestyle that could simultaneously affect a man's fertility and health could explain the identified associations. However, Latif and colleagues[59] examined a large Danish cohort and reported no effect modification based on lifestyle, fertility status, health, and socioeconomic status, suggesting a biological explanation for the association between fertility and hospitalization.

MALE INFERTILITY AND MORTALITY

Given the link between male infertility and chronic disease, researchers have examined the association between infertility and mortality. An analysis of a historic German cohort of 600 men over the span of 35 years failed to establish a relationship between semen quality and mortality, although subgroup analysis suggested a possible association among older members of the cohort.[60] However, given that the study was limited to subjects who lived in post–World War II Germany, the generalizability of the results remains questionable. More recently, Jensen and colleagues[61] evaluated a cohort of more than 43,000 Danish men who had semen analyses performed in the setting of infertility, and found that mortality decreased as sperm concentration increased. Mortality was also found to decrease in a dose-response manner, as sperm motility, morphology, and semen volume increased. A subsequent multicentered American cohort study of more than 11,000 men demonstrated that men with impaired semen parameters (specifically decreased semen volume, sperm concentration, sperm motility, and total sperm count) had significantly higher mortality rates compared with men with normal semen parameters. Specifically, men with 2 or more abnormal semen parameters were found to have a 2.3-fold higher risk of death, although overall incidence of mortality in the study was less than 1%.[62]

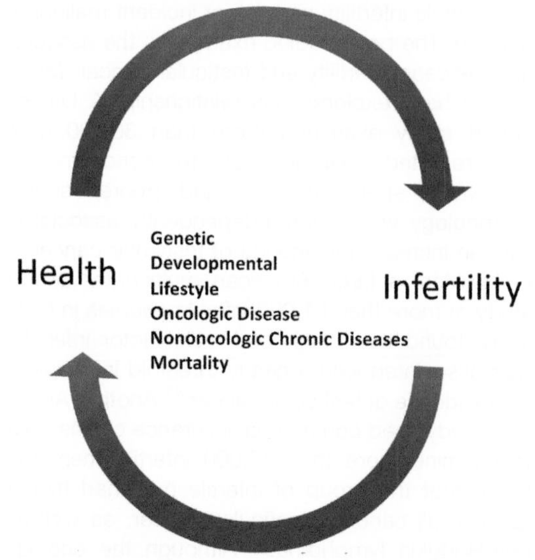

Fig. 1. The relationship between male infertility and overall somatic health.

SUMMARY

A review of the current data suggests that semen quality and male fertility may be a biomarker of overall health (**Fig. 1**). There is a growing body of evidence indicating that male infertility is associated with increased risk of prevalent and incident oncologic, cardiovascular, metabolic, and autoimmune disease, as has also been shown for women. Although the purported associations may arise from genetic, developmental, or lifestyle-based origins, the exact nature of these associations remains unclear. Additional research is required to determine the potential mechanisms and to further clarify the relationship between male infertility and overall health.

DISCLOSURE

The authors have nothing to disclose.

REFERENCES

1. Turp AB, Guler I, Bozkurt N, et al. Infertility and surrogacy first mentioned on a 4000-year-old Assyrian clay tablet of marriage contract in Turkey. Gynecol Endocrinol 2018;34:25–7.
2. Zegers-Hochschild F, Adamson GD, de Mouzon J, et al. International Committee for Monitoring Assisted Reproductive Technology (ICMART) and the World Health Organization (WHO) revised glossary of ART terminology, 2009. Fertil Steril 2009;92:1520–4.
3. Agarwal A, Mulgund A, Hamada A, et al. A unique view on male infertility around the globe. Reprod Biol Endocrinol 2015;13:37.
4. Thoma ME, McLain AC, Louis JF, et al. Prevalence of infertility in the United States as estimated by the current duration approach and a traditional constructed approach. Fertil Steril 2013;99:1324–31.e1.
5. Practice Committee of the American Society for Reproductive Medicine. Diagnostic evaluation of the infertile male: a committee opinion. Fertil Steril 2015;103:e18–25.
6. Salzano A, D'Assante R, Heaney LM, et al. Klinefelter syndrome, insulin resistance, metabolic syndrome, and diabetes: review of literature and clinical perspectives. Endocrine 2018;61(2): 194–203.
7. Weiss JR, Moysich KB, Swede H. Epidemiology of male breast cancer. Cancer Epidemiol Biomarkers Prev 2005;14:20–6.
8. Swerdlow AJ, Schoemaker MJ, Higgins CD, et al. Cancer incidence and mortality in men with Klinefelter syndrome: a cohort study. J Natl Cancer Inst 2005;97:1204–10.
9. Claustres M. Molecular pathology of the CFTR locus in male infertility. Reprod BioMed Online 2005;10: 14–41.
10. Sun F, Turek P, Greene C, et al. Abnormal progression through meiosis in men with nonobstructive azoospermia. Fertil Steril 2007;87:565–71.
11. Paul C, Povey JE, Lawrence NJ, et al. Deletion of genes implicated in protecting the integrity of male germ cells has differential effects on the incidence of DNA breaks and germ cell loss. PLoS One 2007;2:e989.
12. Reitmair AH, Schmits R, Ewel A, et al. MSH2 deficient mice are viable and susceptible to lymphoid tumours. Nat Genet 1995;11:64–70.
13. Li P, Xiao Z, Braciak TA, et al. Systematic immunohistochemical screening for mismatch repair and ERCC1 gene expression from colorectal cancers in China: clinicopathological characteristics and effects on survival. PLoS One 2017;12:e0181615.
14. Zhao L. Mismatch repair protein expression in patients with stage II and III sporadic colorectal cancer. Oncol Lett 2018;15:8053–61.
15. Eisenberg ML, Betts P, Herder D, et al. Increased risk of cancer among azoospermic men. Fertil Steril 2013;100:681–5.
16. Nudell D, Castillo M, Turek PJ, et al. Increased frequency of mutations in DNA from infertile men with meiotic arrest. Hum Reprod 2000;15:1289–94.
17. Stahl PJ, Masson P, Mielnik A, et al. A decade of experience emphasizes that testing for Y microdeletions is essential in American men with azoospermia and severe oligozoospermia. Fertil Steril 2010;94: 1753–6.
18. Jorgez CJ, Weedin JW, Sahin A, et al. Aberrations in pseudoautosomal regions (PARs) found in infertile men with Y-chromosome microdeletions. J Clin Endocrinol Metab 2011;96:E674–9.
19. Garcia Rodriguez A, de la Casa M, Johnston S, et al. Association of polymorphisms in genes coding for antioxidant enzymes and human male infertility. Ann Hum Genet 2019;83:63–72.
20. Ben Rhouma M, Okutman O, Muller J, et al. Genetic aspects of male infertility: from bench to clinic. Gynecol Obstet Fertil Senol 2019;47:54–62 [in French].
21. Barker DJ. The developmental origins of adult disease. J Am Coll Nutr 2004;23:588S–95S.
22. Calkins K, Devaskar SU. Fetal origins of adult disease. Curr Probl Pediatr Adolesc Health Care 2011;41:158–76.
23. Skakkebaek NE, Rajpert-De Meyts E, Main KM. Testicular dysgenesis syndrome: an increasingly common developmental disorder with environmental aspects. Hum Reprod 2001;16:972–8.
24. Skakkebaek NE, Rajpert-De Meyts E, Buck Louis GM, et al. Male reproductive disorders and fertility trends: influences of environment and genetic susceptibility. Physiol Rev 2016;96:55–97.
25. Bang JK, Lyu SW, Choi J, et al. Does infertility treatment increase male reproductive tract disorder? Urology 2013;81:644–8.

26. Posod A, Odri Komazec I, Kager K, et al. Former very preterm infants show an unfavorable cardiovascular risk profile at a preschool age. PLoS One 2016; 11:e0168162.
27. Bloomfield FH. Impact of prematurity for pancreatic islet and beta cell development. J Endocrinol 2018;238(3):R161–71.
28. Belva F, Bonduelle M, Roelants M, et al. Semen quality of young adult ICSI offspring: the first results. Hum Reprod 2016;31:2811–20.
29. Pastuszak AW, Herati AS, Eisenberg ML, et al. The risk of birth defects is not associated with semen parameters or mode of conception in offspring of men visiting a reproductive health clinic. Hum Reprod 2019;34:733–9.
30. Sermondade N, Faure C, Fezeu L, et al. BMI in relation to sperm count: an updated systematic review and collaborative meta-analysis. Hum Reprod Update 2013;19:221–31.
31. Zhang J, Yang B, Cai Z, et al. The negative impact of higher body mass index on sperm quality and erectile function: a cross-sectional study among Chinese males of infertile couples. Am J Mens Health 2019; 13. 1557988318822572.
32. Li Y, Lin H, Li Y, et al. Association between sociopsycho-behavioral factors and male semen quality: systematic review and meta-analyses. Fertil Steril 2011;95:116–23.
33. Jensen TK, Swan S, Jorgensen N, et al. Alcohol and male reproductive health: a cross-sectional study of 8344 healthy men from Europe and the USA. Hum Reprod 2014;29:1801–9.
34. Jensen TK, Hjollund NH, Henriksen TB, et al. Does moderate alcohol consumption affect fertility? Follow up study among couples planning first pregnancy. BMJ 1998;317:505–10.
35. Salonia A, Matloob R, Gallina A, et al. Are infertile men less healthy than fertile men? Results of a prospective case-control survey. Eur Urol 2009;56:1025–31.
36. Shiraishi K, Matsuyama H. Effects of medical comorbidity on male infertility and comorbidity treatment on spermatogenesis. Fertil Steril 2018;110:1006–11.e2.
37. Abdel-Naser MB, Altenburg A, Zouboulis CC, et al. Schistosomiasis (bilharziasis) and male infertility. Andrologia 2019;51:e13165.
38. Moghimi M, Zabihi-Mahmoodabadi S, Kheirkhah-Vakilabad A, et al. Significant correlation between high-risk HPV DNA in semen and impairment of sperm quality in infertile men. Int J Fertil Steril 2019;12:306–9.
39. Trottmann M, Becker AJ, Stadler T, et al. Semen quality in men with malignant diseases before and after therapy and the role of cryopreservation. Eur Urol 2007;52:355–67.
40. Jacobsen R, Bostofte E, Engholm G, et al. Risk of testicular cancer in men with abnormal semen characteristics: cohort study. BMJ 2000;321:789–92.
41. Walsh TJ, Croughan MS, Schembri M, et al. Increased risk of testicular germ cell cancer among infertile men. Arch Intern Med 2009;169: 351–6.
42. Eisenberg ML, Li S, Brooks JD, et al. Increased risk of cancer in infertile men: analysis of U.S. claims data. J Urol 2015;193:1596–601.
43. Walsh TJ, Schembri M, Turek PJ, et al. Increased risk of high-grade prostate cancer among infertile men. Cancer 2010;116:2140–7.
44. Hanson HA, Anderson RE, Aston KI, et al. Subfertility increases risk of testicular cancer: evidence from population-based semen samples. Fertil Steril 2016; 105:322–8.e1.
45. Ruhayel Y, Giwercman A, Ulmert D, et al. Male infertility and prostate cancer risk: a nested case-control study. Cancer Causes Control 2010;21:1635–43.
46. Hanson BM, Eisenberg ML, Hotaling JM. Male infertility: a biomarker of individual and familial cancer risk. Fertil Steril 2018;109:6–19.
47. Anderson RE, Hanson HA, Patel DP, et al. Cancer risk in first- and second-degree relatives of men with poor semen quality. Fertil Steril 2016;106: 731–8.
48. Anderson RE, Hanson HA, Lowrance WT, et al. Childhood cancer risk in the siblings and cousins of men with poor semen quality. J Urol 2017;197: 898–905.
49. Guo D, Li S, Behr B, et al. Hypertension and male fertility. World J Mens Health 2017;35:59–64.
50. Eisenberg ML, Park Y, Hollenbeck AR, et al. Fatherhood and the risk of cardiovascular mortality in the NIH-AARP Diet and Health Study. Hum Reprod 2011;26:3479–85.
51. Eisenberg ML, Li S, Cullen MR, et al. Increased risk of incident chronic medical conditions in infertile men: analysis of United States claims data. Fertil Steril 2016;105:629–36.
52. Wang NN, Dallas K, Li S, et al. The association between varicocoeles and vascular disease: an analysis of U.S. claims data. Andrology 2018;6:99–103.
53. Schisterman EF, Mumford SL, Chen Z, et al. Lipid concentrations and semen quality: the LIFE study. Andrology 2014;2:408–15.
54. Bener A, Al-Ansari AA, Zirie M, et al. Is male fertility associated with type 2 diabetes mellitus? Int Urol Nephrol 2009;41:777–84.
55. Glazer CH, Tottenborg SS, Giwercman A, et al. Male factor infertility and risk of multiple sclerosis: a register-based cohort study. Mult Scler 2018; 24(14):1835–42.
56. Brubaker WD, Li S, Baker LC, et al. Increased risk of autoimmune disorders in infertile men: analysis of US claims data. Andrology 2018;6:94–8.
57. Ortona E, Pierdominici M, Maselli A, et al. Sex-based differences in autoimmune diseases. Ann Ist Super Sanita 2016;52:205–12.

58. Latif T, Kold Jensen T, Mehlsen J, et al. Semen quality as a predictor of subsequent morbidity: a Danish Cohort Study of 4,712 men with long-term follow-up. Am J Epidemiol 2017;186:910–7.
59. Latif T, Lindahl-Jacobsen R, Mehlsen J, et al. Semen quality associated with subsequent hospitalizations - Can the effect be explained by socio-economic status and lifestyle factors? Andrology 2018;6(3):428–35.
60. Groos S, Krause W, Mueller UO. Men with subnormal sperm counts live shorter lives. Soc Biol 2006;53:46–60.
61. Jensen TK, Jacobsen R, Christensen K, et al. Good semen quality and life expectancy: a cohort study of 43,277 men. Am J Epidemiol 2009;170:559–65.
62. Eisenberg ML, Li S, Behr B, et al. Semen quality, infertility and mortality in the USA. Hum Reprod 2014;29:1567–74.

Transgenerational Epigenetics
A Window into Paternal Health Influences on Offspring

Mathew M. Grover, Timothy G. Jenkins, PhD*

KEYWORDS

• DNA methylation • Transgenerational inheritance • Histone modifications • RNA • Sperm
• Paternal age effect

KEY POINTS

- Sperm epigenetics is modifiable over the lifespan of an individual and is impacted by lifestyle decisions, diet, and exposures.
- Sperm epigenetic alterations are capable of altering fertility and offspring phenotype.
- Epigenetics modifications in the paternal germ line has the potential to positively influence offspring phenotype and overall fitness.

INTRODUCTION

The sperm epigenome is deeply important because of its potential effects on intergenerational (1 generation) and transgenerational (2 or more generations) trait inheritance, fertility, and its role in embryonic development.

Over a 50-year period in the latter half of the 20th century, fertility rates decreased significantly. In fact, the average sperm count decrease by more than 41% over that time, and the average seminal volume decreased from 3.4 to 2.75 mL.[1] This trend has continued since then and has begun to raise serious concerns in the health industry. Many factors negatively influence semen quality, such as smoking, age, and obesity, and a somewhat recently explored and powerful force, aberrant sperm epigenetics, may play a role in the negative impact of these signals on sperm function, fertility, and offspring health.[2,3] Although not considered to be independently causative of these fertility deficits, many studies suggest that perturbed epigenetic profiles in sperm contribute to infertility phenotypes, poor embryo quality, and even offspring abnormalities.[4–6]

The reproductive impacts of various toxicants or exposures vary greatly between men and women. In contrast with females, and with some exceptions, males generally do not become entirely infertile when exposed to toxins or as a result of aging, but instead display decreased fertility. This means that they can potentially parent children at older ages or after various exposure types when females may not have this same capacity. This fact often causes clinicians to overlook male fertility as a small barrier to pregnancy and focus on the sometimes absolute barriers to pregnancy that can occur in females. Although justified based on pregnancy data, there are consequences in pursuing this focused approach to fertility care. When taking into consideration the fact that men remain competent to father children despite advanced age or extreme environmental exposures along with recently discovered evidence demonstrating that age and environmental influences can cause significant changes in the

Department of Physiology and Developmental Biology, Brigham Young University, 4005 Life Sciences Building, Provo, UT 84602-5255, USA
* Corresponding author.
E-mail address: Tim_jenkins@byu.edu

Urol Clin N Am 47 (2020) 219–225
https://doi.org/10.1016/j.ucl.2019.12.010

heritable sperm epigenome, these facts reason that men have a great capacity to pass on environmentally influenced characteristics. In short, the fact that a man's fertility is robust over time and after various exposures does not mean that their ability to father healthy children is constant or unaffected. In reality, the fact that men can father children at very old ages or after years of exposures makes men more likely to impact the offspring's health. As a result, it is important to define the impact of various modifiers and what those modifications are capable of inducing in the offspring.

Indeed, studies have shown that epigenetic inheritance can occur via sperm through ancestral exposures, having a proven impact on offspring phenotype.[7–13] These exposures (including toxins or metabolic variations) and subsequent inheritance patters challenge anti-Lamarckian dogma that assumes changes caused by random mutations accumulate over many generations that ultimately lead to a change in a population. Instead, these patterns look more like the inheritance of acquired traits that Lamarck described, and are handed down in distinct ways. The first is through DNA methylation alterations in the paternal genome. DNA methylation (the addition of a methyl group to cytosines in the genome) has the capacity to impact gene transcription through hypermethylation and or hypomethylation at gene promoters which inhibits or facilitates access of transcriptional machinery to the gene promoter.[14] This modification directly on the DNA acts almost like molecular memory that can be passed on to the offspring at certain locations throughout the genome. The second is through RNA and RNA fragments that are found in or on the mature sperm. One study demonstrated this process by inoculating normal oocytes with sperm RNA fragments from mice given a high-fat diet; the metabolic functions of the pups were impaired.[15]

The sperm epigenome also affects the developing embryo. One study showed that global increases in sperm DNA methylation were associated with higher rates of infertility.[16] Thus, a normal sperm epigenome in general is recognized as important to fecundity, whereas abnormal methylation in sperm DNA is associated with infertility and poor outcomes in the offspring. Moreover, when mouse sperm DNA was deliberately hypomethylated through inhibition of the DNA methyltransferase proteins, similar outcomes was seen.[17]

In all, although just one of many influences, the sperm epigenome plays an important part in male fertility and it also seems to be important in the inheritance of acquired traits. This article focuses on the data that support this assertion.

TRANSGENERATIONAL INHERITANCE

Multiple studies demonstrate that male preconception lifestyle decisions have the potential to impact their offspring, for better or worse. Multiple epidemiologic studies have shown deleterious impacts on the offspring after exposure to various chemicals, cigarette smoke, and advancing age in men, to name a few. These troubling findings need to be more thoroughly understood, although promising headway is being made to address the issue at hand.

The recent interest in transgenerational epigenetic inheritance has driven a great deal of research addressing the impact of multiple modifiers (environmental toxins, drugs, lifestyle decisions, diet, aging, etc) of sperm epigenetic signatures and the downstream impact of these changes. This effort has reveled some interesting patterns and potential mechanisms of nongenetic inheritance that seem to fall into 2 distinct categories, either programmatic or disruptive. Examples of programmatic changes to gametes during an individual's life span are those that have the potential to alter the offspring's phenotype in a manner that makes the offspring more competent to respond to some environmental condition. In contrast, disruptive mechanisms of epigenetic inheritance are those that result from exposure to various toxins, environmental pollutants, or the aging process that leads to perturbed offspring phenotypes. Interestingly, these disruptive modifications often result in common abnormalities in the offspring such as neuropsychiatric disease, increased cancer susceptibility, and so on, regardless of the type of insult (aging, cigarette smoke, etc).

The mechanism(s) that account for transgenerational or intergenerational inheritance of specific alterations is not known, although interesting findings are accumulating quickly in the literature. It is likely that the etiology of the inheritance patterns may be unique between programmatic and disruptive transgenerational and intergenerational inheritance. Despite our lack of knowledge regarding the specific patterns of inheritance, it is clear that this phenomenon exists and that it has a significant, but often subtle, impact on the offspring. This finding is particularly true when considering the population wide shifts in cultural or societal activities (changes in diet, stress levels, age at conception, etc).

TWO SUBCATEGORIES OF EPIGENETIC INHERITANCE: PROGRAMMED AND DISRUPTIVE

Some of the earliest examples of potential epigenetic inheritance (and specifically transgenerational inheritance) occurred in Scandinavia. Life for residents of Overkalix, a rural town in far Northern Sweden, in the 1800s was, like most small communities, heavily reliant on crop success to feed the populous. Unfortunately, there was a great deal of variation in the early 1800s in crop success, with multiple famines followed by periods of overabundance. This change in nutrition over a short period of time for a relatively isolated population has provided some of the most important epidemiologic data to date establishing patterns of nongenetic inheritance and has given rise to the interest in epigenetics and transgenerational inheritance that we see today. In fact, a great deal of the most alarming data regarding transgenerational inheritance has arisen from large-scale epidemiologic studies that have shown primarily deleterious impacts on the offspring as a result of environmental exposures in fathers and even in grandfathers.

One of the earliest reports that came from the Overkalix dataset suggested that boys who were 9 to 12 years of age during times with surplus food supplies in Overkalix had grandsons with a decreased lifespans compared with controls.[18] Interestingly, these same individuals, the grandsons of paternal grandfathers who were exposed to food surpluses, had increased mortalities from metabolic (diabetes) and cardiovascular disease.[19] Importantly, although a response from the father to the son (intergenerational inheritance) was observed (even after correction for early social circumstances), the impact of paternal grandfather nutrition remained the most impactful influence on longevity in these individuals.[20]

With these initial Swedish famine studies as a backdrop, investigators began exploring the impact of certain epigenetic modifiers with a specific emphasis on sperm epigenetic modifications and their downstream impact. As described, it seem that, from the growing body of literature, the impacts on offspring or grand offspring will fall largely into 2 categories, either being disruptive in the offspring or programmatic/advantageous.

Disruptive Heritability Patterns

The data that suggest that some intergenerational or transgenerational inheritance patterns are disruptive come in multiple forms. Some of the earliest studies have been focused on epidemiologic data, but new studies using both animal models and humans exist as well. We briefly describe a few examples of disruptive inheritance patterns with aging, obesity and diet, and cigarette exposure in fathers. We discuss the impact of these signals on the gametes as well as on the offspring where data are available.

Studies involving aging and reproduction rarely focus on the male partner. Because female age causes such a striking and absolute barrier to pregnancy, physicians are often more concerned with female age than with male partner age. There is justification in the literature to take this approach, but new and emerging studies available to us now would argue that the male partner should not be ignored. In fact, there is ample evidence in the literature that, as a father advances in age, the likelihood of their offspring developing a neuropsychiatric disorder (autism, schizophrenia, bipolar disease) is significantly increased.[21–26] Not only does this seem to occur from father to son, but 1 recent study has even described an increased incidence of autism in the offspring of older paternal grandfathers (a true transgenerational inheritance pattern).[27] These epidemiologic data opened the door to multiple studies in human and animal models. Smith and colleagues[28] demonstrated in mice that a similar phenotype exists in the offspring sired by older males, namely, that there is a decrease in social and exploratory behaviors the offspring of older males. Our work in human has also shown epigenetic patterns in the sperm that are impacted by age. We identified more than 100 regions in human sperm that have altered DNA methylation patterns as a result of aging.[29] These patterns are particularly interesting when taking into account their enrichment at genomic loci containing genes that have been implicated in schizophrenia and bipolar disorder. Interestingly, these alterations are so consistent that they were used by our laboratory to construct a germline age calculator that can use sperm methylation data to predict an individual's age with a high degree of accuracy.[30] Despite these intriguing findings, there are no analyses in the offspring of these individuals to truly confirm that the methylation alterations could be playing a role in the transmission of this effect over multiple generations. This circumstance is due to the nature of such a study in humans. However, there is a study performed Milekic and colleagues[31] in mice that seems to confirm that such transmission is possible in the context of aging in mammals. Milekic's group confirmed in mice the data previously produced that suggested there is an increase in behavioral abnormalities consistent with common neuropsychiatric disorders in the offspring of older male mice. Not only this, but they were able to identify DNA methylation alterations in the sperm of older fathers, similar to those identified in our human work, while also confirming altered DNA methylation and gene expression in the offspring.

Studies regarding the impact of paternal diet and obesity on offspring phenotype are also available and provide interesting insight into these unique patterns of inheritance. In 1 study in rats, it was found that males exposed to a high -fat diet had offspring and grand offspring with metabolic disorders and decreased insulin sensitivity.[32] Another study has shown that obesity alone in adult male mice could result in altered sperm epigenetic profiles as well as offspring phenotypic changes that persisted over at least 2 generations. The offspring of these obese males had increased adiposity and altered metabolism, and were also obese.[33] In humans, obese men have been shown to have DNA methylation alterations at specific loci in the sperm. In 1 study, these alterations were seen at imprinted genes.[34] Another study in morbidly obese patients sought to understand the reversibility of these alterations with the intervention of bariatric surgery. These patients had significant alterations in their sperm methylome before surgery and almost immediately after surgery there was a dramatic reprogramming of the sperm epigenome.[34] Among the most interesting studies of the heritability of obesity-related alterations to the sperm epigenome and associations to offspring health in humans to date was work that screened newborns who were fathered by obese men. These offspring had alterations in DNA methylation at the IGF2 locus, suggesting that there is some downstream impact of paternal obesity.

Of additional interest to the community is smoking and its impact on sperm DNA methylation and offspring phenotypes and disease susceptibility. In humans, our group has identified distinct genomic loci that have significant DNA methylation alterations in smokers.[35] However, it was not determined what the downstream impact of these alterations may be. Importantly, previous data have demonstrated the preconception cigarette smoking in men is associated with a variety of health consequences in the offspring, including an increased risk of cancers, aneuploidies, and birth defects. One such study showed that the offspring of fathers who smoke (before conception), coupled with mothers who do not, have an increased chance of being diagnosed with a variety of childhood cancers, including cancers blood and nervous system tumors.[36] Very recently, a group in Cost Rica identified an increased risk of leukemia in the offspring of fathers who consumed cigarette smoke before conception.[37] Additional studies in human sperm have identified alterations to important chromatin structures in the sperm of smokers.[38] One interesting study showed that male mice exposed to nicotine fathered offspring that had altered behavioral phenotypes over 2 generations. Specifically, it was found that the offspring of males exposed to nicotine had a decreased capacity for learning and attention and increased locomotor activity.

Although these studies represent only a small portion of the data that are available regarding the potentially disruptive nature of transgenerational inheritance, they clearly demonstrate that what the father does actually matters. Preconception lifestyle decisions and exposure to various modifiers places the offspring at significantly increased risk of various abnormalities.

Programmatic Heritability Patterns

Although many studies have shown that the impacts of a father's lifestyle decisions and exposures can result in metabolic disorders and an increased risk of various diseases, it is clear that some signals carried from parent to offspring in a nongenetic fashion are of a different type. Some even seem to be beneficial to the offspring, as if the gamete had the capacity to inform the offspring of some environmental condition and prepare them to cope with it in a unique way. The mechanisms that underlie this process are poorly understood and quite controversial, but great strides are being made at a rapid pace.

Perhaps one of the most dramatic displays of what seems to be a programmed inheritance of acquired traits was displayed in a study published in 2014 in *Nature Neuroscience*.[39] The authors of this study wanted to explore the impact of fear conditioning in male mice and determine if this conditioning could somehow impact the offspring. The study involved the scent acetophenone (an aromatic ketone commonly used in perfumes) and an electric shock. In brief, male mice were exposed to the scent while simultaneously being exposed to a gentle shock on their foot pads. The animals soon became conditioned to the smell and associated it with the shock and were startled each time the odor was introduced, regardless of the presence of an associated shock. These F0 animals were humanely killed and the sperm that were extracted were either used to generate new offspring or to perform DNA methylation analysis. Intriguingly, the offspring of males exposed to the shock would respond similarly to the odor. Specifically, they would display the startled phenotype when exposed to acetophenone unlike the control group, whose fathers were not exposed to the scent and subsequent shock. Further, the offspring of exposed males also had a higher sensitivity to acetophenone (they were able to identify the scent at lower concentrations).

Taken together, the offspring of males conditioned to the acetophenone scent with associated shock were afraid of this scent when it was detected. The authors of the study attempted to explore the mechanism by which this environmental queue was passed on the offspring. It was found that there was significantly altered methylation in the sperm of the males exposed to acetophenone and shock at the odor receptor gene Olfr151 (the receptor known to bind acetophenone). The authors propose that this is the method by which signals are handed down to the offspring.

To highlight the unique nature of each inheritance pattern (and the fact that they all do not necessarily fit neatly into either the programmatic inheritance category or the disruptive inheritance category), it is important to site additional work performed on nicotine. We mentioned a study elsewhere in this article with largely negative consequences on the offspring. However, other authors have also assessed the intergenerational inheritance patterns associated with paternal nicotine exposure and have identified some interesting findings that suggest there may be some more programmatic like responses by the offspring. In a recent publication from Oliver Rando's laboratory at the University of Massachusetts, they describe how paternal exposure of nicotine induced protective responses (a decreased sensitivity) in the offspring.[40] They found that the offspring of male mice exposed to nicotine could survive high levels of nicotine exposure; in the most extreme case, the animals were able to survive toxic levels of nicotine injection. This finding suggests that the offspring of nicotine-exposed males were desensitized to the drug by a still unknown mechanism.

Although many more studies exist that demonstrate the impact of transgenerational inheritance, these studies highlight what is known in the field today. The 2 studies that seem to suggest that the sperm are able to orient the offspring to a specific environment are remarkable. This finding truly does fly in the face of traditional thinking regarding the inheritance of traits through Darwinian natural selection, but may offer potential new avenues of exploration that will impact many fields from evolution to medicine.

SUMMARY

It is essential to understand the consequences of our decisions, particularly when those consequences can affect others. It is only recently that we have learned about the impacts of a father's preconception lifestyle decisions and exposures on their offspring. Although there remains a great deal of work that must be done to fully understand the mechanisms that underlie the process and the full impact these mechanism will have on the offspring, we must to not ignore what has already been demonstrated. These patterns of nongenetic inheritance of acquired characteristics have fundamentally changed the way that we think about the inheritance of traits and, in the future, we may be able to identify patterns in the sperm that are predictive of outcomes in the offspring such that we can generate highly personalized approaches to reproductive care. In an older male who wishes to father a child, for example, we may be able to help offer a precise probability of him having a child with a specific neuropsychiatric disease as a result of the work that is being performed today. There is a great deal that still needs to be explored and determined, but the potential impact of this work in the clinic and in our understanding basic biological principles is very significant.

DISCLOSURE

M.M. Grover has nothing to report. T.G. Jenkins is a share holder in Inherent Biosciences (an epigenetics company) and Nanonc (a microfluidics company specializing in sperm isolation).

REFERENCES

1. Carlsen E, Giwercman A, Keiding N, et al. Evidence for decreasing quality of semen during past 50 years. BMJ 1992;305(6854):609–13.
2. Dai JB, Wang ZX, Qiao ZD. The hazardous effects of tobacco smoking on male fertility. Asian J Androl 2015;17(6):954–60.
3. Palmer NO, Bakos HW, Fullston T, et al. Impact of obesity on male fertility, sperm function and molecular composition. Spermatogenesis 2012;2(4):253–63.
4. Jenkins TG, Carrell DT. The sperm epigenome and potential implications for the developing embryo. Reproduction 2012;143(6):727–34.
5. Jenkins TG, Aston KI, Meyer TD, et al. Decreased fecundity and sperm DNA methylation patterns. Fertil Steril 2016;105(1):51–7.e1-3.
6. Aston KI, Uren PJ, Jenkins TG, et al. Aberrant sperm DNA methylation predicts male fertility status and embryo quality. Fertil Steril 2015;104(6):1388–97.e1-5.
7. Carone BR, Fauquier L, Habib N, et al. Paternally induced transgenerational environmental reprogramming of metabolic gene expression in mammals. Cell 2010;143(7):1084–96.
8. Govorko D, Bekdash RA, Zhang C, et al. Male germline transmits fetal alcohol adverse effect on

hypothalamic proopiomelanocortin gene across generations. Biol Psychiatry 2012;72(5):378–88.
9. Kohli A, Garcia MA, Miller RL, et al. Secondhand smoke in combination with ambient air pollution exposure is associated with increased CpG methylation and decreased expression of IFN-gamma in T effector cells and Foxp3 in T regulatory cells in children. Clin Epigenetics 2012;4(1):17.
10. Bosse Y, Postma DS, Sin DD, et al. Molecular signature of smoking in human lung tissues. Cancer Res 2012;72(15):3753–63.
11. Word B, Lyn-Cook LE Jr, Mwamba B, et al. Cigarette smoke condensate induces differential expression and promoter methylation profiles of critical genes involved in lung cancer in NL-20 Lung cells in vitro: short-term and chronic exposure. Int J Toxicol 2013;32(1):23–31.
12. Knezovich JG, Ramsay M. The effect of preconception paternal alcohol exposure on epigenetic remodeling of the h19 and rasgrf1 imprinting control regions in mouse offspring. Front Genet 2012;3:10.
13. Liang F, Diao L, Liu J, et al. Paternal ethanol exposure and behavioral abnormities in offspring: associated alterations in imprinted gene methylation. Neuropharmacology 2014;81:126–33.
14. Navarro-Costa P, Nogueira P, Carvalho M, et al. Incorrect DNA methylation of the DAZL promoter CpG island associates with defective human sperm. Hum Reprod 2010;25(10):2647–54.
15. Chen Q, Yan W, Duan E. Epigenetic inheritance of acquired traits through sperm RNAs and sperm RNA modifications. Nat Rev Genet 2016;17(12):733–43.
16. Benchaib M, Braun V, Ressnikof D, et al. Influence of global sperm DNA methylation on IVF results. Hum Reprod 2005;20(3):768–73.
17. Li E, Bestor TH, Jaenisch R. Targeted mutation of the DNA methyltransferase gene results in embryonic lethality. Cell 1992;69(6):915–26.
18. Bygren LO, Kaati G, Edvinsson S. Longevity determined by paternal ancestors' nutrition during their slow growth period. Acta Biotheor 2001;49(1):53–9.
19. Kaati G, Bygren LO, Edvinsson S. Cardiovascular and diabetes mortality determined by nutrition during parents' and grandparents' slow growth period. Eur J Hum Genet 2002;10(11):682–8.
20. Kaati G, Bygren LO, Pembrey M, et al. Transgenerational response to nutrition, early life circumstances and longevity. Eur J Hum Genet 2007;15(7):784–90.
21. Foldi CJ, Eyles DW, Flatscher-Bader T, et al. New perspectives on rodent models of advanced paternal age: relevance to autism. Front Behav Neurosci 2011;5:32.
22. Idring S, Magnusson C, Lundberg M, et al. Parental age and the risk of autism spectrum disorders: findings from a Swedish population-based cohort. Int J Epidemiol 2014;43(1):107–15.
23. Dalman C. Advanced paternal age increases risk of bipolar disorder in offspring. Evid Based Ment Health 2009;12(2):59.
24. Kuratomi G, Iwamoto K, Bundo M, et al. Aberrant DNA methylation associated with bipolar disorder identified from discordant monozygotic twins. Mol Psychiatry 2008;13(4):429–41.
25. Miller B, Messias E, Miettunen J, et al. Meta-analysis of paternal age and schizophrenia risk in male versus female offspring. Schizophr Bull 2011;37(5):1039–47.
26. Naserbakht M, Ahmadkhaniha HR, Mokri B, et al. Advanced paternal age is a risk factor for schizophrenia in Iranians. Ann Gen Psychiatry 2011;10:15.
27. Frans EM, Sandin S, Reichenberg A, et al. Autism risk across generations: a population-based study of advancing grandpaternal and paternal age. JAMA Psychiatry 2013;70(5):516–21.
28. Smith RG, Kember RL, Mill J, et al. Advancing paternal age is associated with deficits in social and exploratory behaviors in the offspring: a mouse model. PLoS One 2009;4(12):e8456.
29. Jenkins TG, Aston KI, Pflueger C, et al. Age-associated sperm DNA methylation alterations: possible implications in offspring disease susceptibility. PLoS Genet 2014;10(7):e1004458.
30. Jenkins TG, Aston KI, Cairns B, et al. Paternal germ line aging: DNA methylation age prediction from human sperm. BMC Genomics 2018;19(1):763.
31. Milekic MH, Xin Y, O'Donnell A, et al. Age-related sperm DNA methylation changes are transmitted to offspring and associated with abnormal behavior and dysregulated gene expression. Mol Psychiatry 2015;20(8):995–1001.
32. de Castro Barbosa T, Ingerslev LR, Alm PS, et al. High-fat diet reprograms the epigenome of rat spermatozoa and transgenerationally affects metabolism of the offspring. Mol Metab 2016;5(3):184–97.
33. Fullston T, Ohlsson Teague EM, Palmer NO, et al. Paternal obesity initiates metabolic disturbances in two generations of mice with incomplete penetrance to the F2 generation and alters the transcriptional profile of testis and sperm microRNA content. FASEB J 2013;27(10):4226–43.
34. Soubry A, Guo L, Huang Z, et al. Obesity-related DNA methylation at imprinted genes in human sperm: results from the TIEGER study. Clin Epigenetics 2016;8:51.
35. Jenkins TG, James ER, Alonso DF, et al. Cigarette smoking significantly alters sperm DNA methylation patterns. Andrology 2017;5(6):1089–99.
36. Ji BT, Shu XO, Linet MS, et al. Paternal cigarette smoking and the risk of childhood cancer among offspring of nonsmoking mothers. J Natl Cancer Inst 1997;89(3):238–44.
37. Frederiksen LE, Erdmann F, Wesseling C, et al. Parental tobacco smoking and risk of childhood

leukemia in Costa Rica: a population-based case-control study. Environ Res 2019;180:108827.
38. Hamad MF, Shelko N, Kartarius S, et al. Impact of cigarette smoking on histone (H2B) to protamine ratio in human spermatozoa and its relation to sperm parameters. Andrology 2014;2(5):666–77.
39. Dias BG, Ressler KJ. Parental olfactory experience influences behavior and neural structure in subsequent generations. Nat Neurosci 2014;17(1):89–96.
40. Vallaster MP, Kukreja S, Bing XY, et al. Paternal nicotine exposure alters hepatic xenobiotic metabolism in offspring. Elife 2017;6 [pii:e24771].

Spermatogonial Stem Cell Culture in Oncofertility

Sherin David, PhD, Kyle E. Orwig, PhD*

KEYWORDS

• Spermatogonial stem cell culture • Fertility preservation • Male fertility

KEY POINTS

- Chemotherapy, radiation, and other medical treatments can cause permanent infertility. Sperm freezing is the standard of care method to preserve male fertility.
- Testicular tissue freezing is an experimental option to preserve the fertility of prepubertal boys and others who cannot produce sperm. Testicular tissues contain spermatogonial stem cells.
- Spermatogonial stem cell–based techniques that are currently in the research pipeline may be available in the male fertility clinic of the future.
- To facilitate clinical translation, methods are needed to isolate and enrich human spermatogonial stem cells as well as expand their numbers in culture.

INTRODUCTION

Advancements in cancer therapies over the past several decades have led to a rise in pediatric cancer survival rates to approximately 88%.[1] This increase in cancer survivorship has made it increasingly important to address factors that affect patient quality of life posttreatment, including treatment-induced gonadotoxicity and increased risk of infertility.[2,3] Most patients who are exposed to gonadotoxic therapies experience transient azoospermia and will recover normal levels of spermatogenesis within 1 to 5 years posttreatment[4]; however, approximately 24% of patients will be rendered permanently infertile by treatment for their primary disease.[5] The extent and permanence of azoospermia depends on a combination of several factors, including the primary disease diagnosis and the therapeutic regimen employed to treat the disease. Methods to predict the risk of infertility are imperfect,[6] but some guidance is available to predict treatment regimens that are associated with significant or high risk of infertility.[7,8] The prospect of having biological children is important to cancer survivors, and the risk of iatrogenic infertility causes psychosocial stress in these individuals.[9] Therefore, the American Society of Clinical Oncology, the American Society for Reproductive Medicine, and the American Academy of Pediatrics recommend that all patients with cancer and patients receiving cytotoxic treatments for hematologic conditions be counseled about the risk of infertility and about methods for fertility preservation before the onset of treatment.[10–13]

The standard of care approach to preserve fertility in adolescent and adult male patients is cryopreservation of spermatozoa that can be used at a later time to establish pregnancy through assisted reproductive technology.[14,15] This option is not available to prepubertal patients who do not produce sperm; however, several centers around the world are cryopreserving testicular tissues for young patients with anticipation that spermatogonial stem cells (SSCs) in those tissues might be used to restore fertility in the future.[16–23]

Department of Obstetrics, Gynecology and Reproductive Sciences, Molecular Genetics and Developmental Biology Graduate Program, Magee-Womens Research Institute, University of Pittsburgh School of Medicine, 204 Craft Avenue, Pittsburgh, PA 15213, USA
* Corresponding author.
E-mail address: orwigke@upmc.edu

Urol Clin N Am 47 (2020) 227–244
https://doi.org/10.1016/j.ucl.2020.01.001

SPERMATOGONIAL STEM CELL TRANSPLANTATION TO RESTORE FERTILITY

Several new technologies have emerged over the past 25 years that may allow patients to use their cryopreserved testicular tissues to produce sperm and have biological offspring, including SSC transplantation, de novo testicular morphogenesis, testicular tissue organ culture, testicular tissue grafting or xenografting, and derivation of germ cells from induced pluripotent stem cells.[24,25] SSC transplantation is a mature technology that may be ready for translation to the male fertility clinic. In fact, Radford and colleagues[26,27] reported a clinical trial in 1999 in which testicular cell suspensions were cryopreserved for 12 patients with Hodgkin disease. Seven of those patients returned to have their cryopreserved cells, including SSCs, transplanted back into their testes via injection into the rete testis space.[27] Although follow-up studies on the outcome of transplantation in those cases have not been reported, the study demonstrates patient willingness to undergo an experimental SSC-based therapy to have a biological child.

Like other tissue-specific stem cells, SSCs have the potential to colonize the testicular niche and regenerate spermatogenesis. Brinster and colleagues[28,29] first demonstrated this principle 25 years ago by showing that mouse testicular cell suspensions containing SSCs could be transplanted into the seminiferous tubules of an infertile mouse recipient to restore complete spermatogenesis and fertility. This method has since been replicated in a number of mammalian species, including rats, sheep, goats, pigs, bulls, dogs, and primates.[30–36] SSCs from all ages, newborn to adult, are competent to regenerate spermatogenesis, and spermatogenesis can be restored from testicular cells that have been cryopreserved for as long as 14 years.[33,37–41] Thus, it appears feasible to cryopreserve testicular tissues/cells containing SSCs for prepubertal patients and recover those cells years later for autologous transplantation and regeneration of spermatogenesis.

Testicular cells are typically transplanted into the recipient testis through the rete testis space that is contiguous with all seminiferous tubules.[33,42–44] SSCs migrate from the lumen of the seminiferous tubules, through the blood-testis barrier (BTB), to the basement membrane. Rac1 and β1 Integrin have been shown to be critical in SSC transmigration through the BTB and attachment to the basement membrane, respectively, in mice.[45,46] Despite innate properties allowing SSCs to penetrate the BTB, most transplanted cells are eliminated through phagocytosis by Sertoli cells, which may be one factor that reduces overall efficiency of the method.[47] Nagano and colleagues[48] evaluated the kinetics of SSC engraftment in the mouse testis and deduced that transplantation with 1 million testicular cells led to colonization and spermatogenesis by 19 SSCs. Thus, methods to isolate and enrich SSCs and expand their numbers in culture are needed to ensure robust engraftment and regeneration of spermatogenesis.

In fertility preservation centers that provide testicular tissue cryopreservation services, approximately 20% of testicular volume from one testis is typically biopsied, although some centers allow for collection of larger volumes and/or biopsy of both testes.[22,23,49] Hence, the number of SSCs obtained from small biopsies of prepubertal testes could be a limiting factor in the successful application SSC transplantation in the clinic. One way to overcome this limitation is to isolate and enrich SSCs from the testicular biopsy and expand their numbers in vitro before transplantation. These approaches might also be used to assess and eliminate malignant contamination, as described in the following section.

SORTING METHODS TO ISOLATE AND ENRICH SPERMATOGONIAL STEM CELLS AS WELL AS ELIMINATE MALIGNANT CONTAMINATION

Using SSC transplantation as a functional assay, several cell surface markers have been identified that are conserved between murine and human spermatogonia. Murine SSCs have been shown to exhibit the phenotype GPR125^{+} (G-protein coupled receptor 125), EpCAM^{low} (epithelial cell adhesion molecule), ITGA6^{+} (α6 integrin), ITGB1^{+} (β1 integrin), CD9^{+}, THY1^{+} (CD90), GFRα1^{+} (GDNF family receptor alpha 1), MCAM^{+} (melanoma cell adhesion molecule 1), ITGAV^{-} (αV integrin), cKIT^{-} (CD117 or stem cell growth factor), MHC-I^{-} (major histocompatibility complex class I), SCA-1^{-} (stem cells antigen 1).[50–58] Characterization of human spermatogonia has identified GPR125, EpCAM, ITGA6, and GFRA1, as well as FGFR3 (fibroblast growth factor receptor 3), SSEA4 (stage specific embryonic antigen 4), TSPAN33 (tetraspanin 33), as cell surface markers of human SSCs.[59–61] In addition to its application in basic research, the ability to identify and enrich SSCs is important for clinical translation of SSC transplantation as a method to restore fertility. These methods could be especially valuable for patients with malignancies that may contaminate testicular cells, posing a risk of reintroducing cancer cells into patient survivors. A study using a rat model showed that transplanting a testicular cell suspension with as few as 20 leukemic cells could cause the disease to recur in the recipient.[62] Some studies have reported the use of multiparametric flow cytometry methods to negatively select spermatogonia from cancer cells.[58,63] Other reports used markers for both spermatogonia and cancer cells for a more stringent segregation of the 2 populations but produced conflicting results.[64–66] In addition, these reports were based on the use of cancer cell lines, and the efficacy of these methods in eliminating heterogeneous populations of malignant cells needs to be determined.

Although sorting techniques to enrich SSCs and eliminate contaminating malignant cells are promising, there is a need to develop stringent methods to test and quantify residual malignant contamination before autologous transplantation. Polymerase chain reaction (PCR)-based methods to detect minimal residual disease may be used in addition to flow cytometry approaches to increase the sensitivity of selection. Currently, there is limited information about how low-level contamination detected by PCR corresponds to tumor-forming capacity and, hence, the absolute risk for inducing relapse remains difficult to predict.[67,68] Development of human SSC culture methods may enable clonal expansion of SSCs from an enriched population providing an extra level of stringency for decontamination of patient samples.[69]

Methods for enriching spermatogonia are routinely used to establish SSC culture (**Table 1**). Shortly after the discovery of the role of glial cell line–derived neurotropic factor (GDNF) on SSC self-renewal,[70] Kanatsu-Shinohara and colleagues[71] described a method for the long-term culture of mouse SSCs. In this report, they placed testicular cells on plates coated with gelatin; the testicular somatic cells selectively adhered to the plates, whereas germ cells remained floating and could be aspirated and plated onto secondary plates. This approach served the dual purpose of enriching SSCs and removing testicular somatic cells that can rapidly overwhelm the cultures. After 2 or more rounds of differential plating, floating cells were plated on mouse embryonic fibroblasts in low serum medium supplemented with epidermal growth factor (EGF), leukemia inhibitory factor (LIF), GDNF, and fibroblast growth factor 2 (FGF2). Subsequent studies used fluorescence-activated cell sorting (FACS) and magnetic-activated cell sorting (MACS) for the cell surface marker, THY1, to enrich spermatogonia.[72–74] Spermatogonial stem cell transplantation provided the experimental evidence that functional rodent SSCs could be maintained with expansion in number during long-term culture.[71,73–76] Cultured SSCs not only regenerated spermatogenesis in infertile recipients, but also produced sperm that were competent to fertilize rodent oocytes and give rise to healthy offspring.[71,73]

HUMAN SPERMATOGONIAL STEM CELL CULTURE: COMPONENTS AND METHODS OF ANALYSIS

In 2009, Sadri-Ardekani and colleagues[18] reported the long-term culture of adult human SSCs following a protocol very similar to that described by Kanatsu-Shinohara and colleagues[71] in their first report on mouse SSC cultures. Specifically, differential plating was used to reduce the number of testicular somatic cells, which attached to the plate; floating germ cells were passaged onto plates coated with human placental laminin in StemPro medium supplemented with EGF, LIF, GDNF, and FGF2. Using this method, the investigators reported that human SSCs could be maintained for several months and expanded more than 18,000-fold.[18] The same group later reported similar success culturing SSCs from prepubertal human testes.[77]

There are now more than 20 reports on human SSC culture (see **Table 1**). Many have used differential plating on plastic, lectin, collagen, or gelatin as the sole means to enrich SSCs and/or reduce testicular somatic cells before culture.[18,77–86] Others have supplemented differential plating with Percoll gradient selection[87,88] and/or positive or negative selection for cell surface markers using FACS or MACS[87,89–93] or used FACS/MACS selection alone.[94,95] Positive selection markers used for human SSC culture have included ITGA6, CD9, GPR125, SSEA4, and EPCAM. Negative selection markers have included cKIT, CD45, and THY1 (see **Table 1**). Interestingly, although THY1 has been used as a positive selection marker before mouse SSC culture,[73] Smith and colleagues[95] used THY1 as a negative marker of human SSCs and in fact used irradiated THY1+ human testis cells as feeders for their human SSC cultures.

Human spermatogonia, like murine spermatogonia, have been shown to require an extracellular matrix (ECM) or feeder-cell–based substrates to promote the attachment, survival, and proliferation in vitro. Feeder cells that have been used to culture human SSCs include fibroblasts derived from human embryonic stem cells, human Sertoli cells, mouse embryonic fibroblasts, mouse endothelial cells, human testicular somatic cells, and THY1+ testicular cells (see **Table 1**).[78–80,88,93–96] ECM

Table 1
Literature review of reports on human SSC culture

Citation	Duration of Culture	Sort/ Differential Plating	Medium	Growth Factors	Feeders or ECM	Passaging Technique	End Point	Type and Age of Donor	Claim
Sadri-Ardekani et al,[18] 2009	15 wk	Differential plating on plastic	MEM+10% FCS for differential plating followed by StemPro-34	20 ng/mL EGF, 10 ng/mL GDNF, 10 ng/mL LIF, 10 ng/mL bFGF	Human placental laminin	Passaged every 7–10 d using Trypsin EDTA and differential passaging if there was somatic cell overgrowth	Xeno transplants; ICC – PLZF; RT-PCR – PLZF, ITGA6, ITGB1;	Adult orchidectomy patients (n = 6)	18,000-fold increase in xeno transplant colonizing activity over 64 d in culture
Wu et al,[78] 2009	1 wk	Differential plating on gelatin	MEMα	20 ng/mL GDNF, 150 ng/mL GFRA1, 1 ng/mL bFGF	C166 mouse endothelial cells	Not reported	ICC – UCHL1	Prepubertal male aged 2–10 y diagnosed with cancer (n = 2)	UCHL1+ spermatogonia can be maintained at least 19 d. No quantification. GDNF required.
Chen et al,[94] 2009	2 mo	MACS for ITGA6	DMEM	10 ng/ml GDNF, 4 ng/ml bFGF, 1500 IU/mL LIF	Human embryonic stem cells derived fibroblasts (hdF)	Passaged every 4–5 d using cell dissociation buffer or trypsin	ICC – OCT4, SSEA1, ITGA6; RT-PCR – OCT4, STRA8, DAZL, NOTCH1, NGN3, SOX3, KIT	Fetal	Colonies maintained over 10 passages. No quantification.

Lim et al,[87] 2010	>6 mo	Percoll selection, differential plating on plastic and collagen followed by MACS for CD9	DMEM during enrichment followed by StemPro-34	10 ng/mL GDNF, 10 ng/mL bFGF, 20 ng/mL EGF, 10,000 U/mL LIF	Laminin	Passaged very 2 wk using Trypsin	RT-PCR - OCT4, ITGA6, ITGB1, cKIT, TH2B, SYCP3, TP-1; MTT; TUNEL; ICC - GFRA1, CD-9, ITGA6; Alkaline phosphatase staining	Males with obstructive and non obstructive azoospermia (n = 37)	Clumps maintained and continued proliferating over 12 passages (>26 wk). Total cells quantified.
He et al,[89] 2010	14 d	Differential plating on plastic and MACS for GFR125	DMEM/F12 during enrichment followed StemPro-34	100 ng/mL GDNF, 300 ng/mL GFRA1-Fc, 10 ng/mL NUDT6, 10 ng/mL LIF, 20 ng/mL EGF, 30 ng/mL TGFB, 100 ng/mL Nodal	0.1% gelatin	Not reported	ICC – GPR125, ITGA6, GFRA1, THY1	Adult organ donors (n = 5)	GPR125+ cells proliferated during 2 wk in culture, but were not quantified.

(*continued on next page*)

Table 1
(*continued*)

Citation	Duration of Culture	Sort/ Differential Plating	Medium	Growth Factors	Feeders or ECM	Passaging Technique	End Point	Type and Age of Donor	Claim
Kokkinaki et al,[90] 2011	4–5 mo	Differential plating on FBS-coated dish, treatment with RBC Lysis Buffer and Dead Cell Removal Kit followed by SSEA4 MACS	StemPro-34	10 ng/mL GDNF, 10 ng/mL bFGF, 20 ng/mL EGF, 10,000 U/mL LIF	Growth factor-reduced matrigel	Passaged manually at 1 mo followed by digestion with dispase + collagenase every 10–15 d	Morphology, number of colonies and cells/colony, RT-PCR for SSC markers (PLZF, GPR125, SSEA4) and pluripotency markers (KLF4, OCT4, LIN28, SOX2, NANOG)	14, 34, and 45-year-old organ donors (n = 3)	Number of colonies and number of cells per colony increased during 5 months in culture.
Sadri-Ardekani et al,[77] 2011	15.5 and 10 wk	Differential plating on plastic	StemPro-34	20 ng/mL EGF, 10 ng/mL GDNF, 10 ng/mL LIF, 10 ng/mL bFGF	Human placental laminin	Passaged every 7–10 d using Trypsin EDTA and differential passaging if there was somatic cell overgrowth	Xeno transplants; RT-PCR – PLZF, ITGA6, ITGB1, CD9, GFRA1, GPR125, UCHL1	Prepuberatal male patients with Hodgkin lymphoma; 6.5 and 8.0 years old (n = 2)	5.6-fold increase in xeno transplant colonizing activity over 14 d in culture and 6.2-fold increase over 21 d in culture.
Nowroozi et al,[79] 2011	18 d	Differential plating on lectin-coated plates	DMEM	Not reported	Human Sertoli cells	Passaged every 7 d with Trypsin EDTA	ICC – OCT4, Vimentin; Alkaline phosphatase staining	Adults with non obstructive azoospermia (n = 47)	Colonies were observed over 18 d in culture. No quantification.

Liu et al,[88] 2011	1 mo	Percoll separation and differential plating on plastic	DMEM/F12	Not reported	Human Sertoli cells	Not reported	ICC – OCT4, SSEA4; Flow cytometry – OCT4	Fetal (n = 5)	OCT4+ cells observed; timeframe uncertain. No quantification.
Mirzapour et al,[80] 2012	5 wk	Differential plating on lectin-coated plates	DMEM	Various concent-rations of bFGF and LIF	Human Sertoli cells	Passaged every 7 d using Trypsin EDTA	Xeno transplants; alkaline phosphatase staining; ICC – OCT4, Vimentin; RT-PCR – OCT4, NANOG, STRA8, PIWIL2, VASA	Adult males with NOA-maturation arrest (n = 20)	Tested bFGF and LIF concentrations. Colony number increased in some conditions over 30 d in culture.
Koruji et al,[86] 2012	2 mo	Differential plating on plastic	DMEM+ 5%FCS	20 ng/mL GDNF, 10 ng/mL bFGF, 10 ng/mL LIF, 20 ng/mL EGF	Laminin or plastic	Passaged every 5–7 d using Trypsin EDTA	Morphology-number and diameter of colonies; RT-PCR – PLZF, DAZL, OCT4, VASA, ITGA6, ITGB1	Adult males with NOA	Clusters present after 2 mo. Xeno transplant colonizing activity and expression of spermatogonial markers reported. No quantification.

(*continued on next page*)

Table 1
(continued)

Citation	Duration of Culture	Sort/ Differential Plating	Medium	Growth Factors	Feeders or ECM	Passaging Technique	End Point	Type and Age of Donor	Claim
Goharbakhsh et al,[81] 2013	52 d	Differential plating on plastic for cells $>10^6$, all cells were plated is number$<10^6$	DMEM-F12	10 ng/mL GDNF, 10 ng/mL bFGF, 20 ng/mL EGF, 10,000 U/mL LIF	20 μL/mL laminin or 0.2% gelatin	Passaged every 7–10 d, method was not mentioned	Morphologic observation of EB-like colonies and ICC staining for GPR125	Azoospermic adult males (n = 12)	Clusters observed over several passages during 52 d in culture. GPR125+ cells observed at end of culture. No quantification of clusters or GPR125 cells.
Piravar et al,[82] 2013	6 wk	Differential plating on plastic	DMEM/F12 for 16 h then StemPro-34	10 ng/mL GDNF, 20 ng/mL EGF, 10 ng/mL LIF	Uncoated plates for the first 14 d followed by laminin	Trypsinization every 2 wk	qPCR for UCHL1	Non obstructive azoospermic males (n = 10)	Clusters number increased over 6-wk of culture. UCHL1 expression observed by RT-PCR.
Akhondi, MM et al,[112] 2013	6 wk	Enrichment was not performed	StemPro-34	10 ng/mL GDNF, 20 ng/mL EGF, 10 ng/mL LIF	Not reported	Trypsinization every 10 d	ICC for Oct4; qPCR for PLZF	44-year-old organ donor (n = 1)	Cluster number increased during 6-wk culture. OCT4 observed by ICC at end of culture. PLZF expression observed by RT-PCR

Zheng et al,[83] 2014	2 wk	Differential plating on plastic and collagen	DMEM during enrichment followed by StemPro-34	20 ng/mL EGF, 10 ng/mL GDNF, 10 ng/mL LIF, 10 ng/mL bFGF	Not reported	Passaged using Trypsin when confluent	Flow cytometry - SSEA4; qRT-PCR - UTF1, FGFR3, SALL4, PLZF, DAZL, VIM, ACTA2, GATA4	Adult organ donors (n = 8)	SSEA4+ spermatogonia decreased over time in culture. VIM+, ACTA2+ somatic cells were the main cell type present after 48 d in culture
Chikhovskaya et al,[91] 2014	2 wk	Differential plating on plastic followed by MACS for ITGA6 and differential plating on Collagen I and Laminin	StemPro-34	20 ng/mL EGF, 10 ng/mL GDNF, 10 ng/mL LIF, 10 ng/mL bFGF	MEFs or plastic	Not reported	qPCR for PLZF, MAGEA4, CD49f, DAZL, UTF1, DDX4, TM4SF1, ACTA2; flow cytometry for SSEA4, CD29, CD44, CD49f, CD73, CD90, CD105, HLAABC, HLADR, CD31, CD34, CD117, CD133	Adult patients with cancer undergoing bilateral orchidectomy (n = 3)	Mixed cultures: rapid proliferation of testicular somatic cells and rapid decrease in PLZF+ and MAGEA4+ germ cells. Isolated spermatogonia degenerated by 2 wk in culture.

(*continued on next page*)

Table 1
(continued)

Citation	Duration of Culture	Sort/ Differential Plating	Medium	Growth Factors	Feeders or ECM	Passaging Technique	End Point	Type and Age of Donor	Claim
Smith et al,[95] 2014	21 d	FACS – CD45-, THY1-, SSEA4+	StemPro-34	20 ng/mL EGF, 10 ng/mL GDNF, 10 ng/mL LIF, 10 ng/mL bFGF	Adult human THY1+ cells	Not reported	ICC – SSEA4, VASA	Adults with normal spermatogenesis (n = 13)	Colonies expressing SSEA4 and VASA were present at 21 d. No quantification.
Guo et al,[92] 2015	2 mo	Differential plating on plastic with DMEM-F12 followed by MACS for GPR125	StemPro-34	20 ng/mL EGF, 10 ng/mL bFGF, 10 ng/mL LIF, 50 ng/mL GDNF	Hydrogel Stem Easy	Not reported	Morphologic observation; cell proliferation assay; ICC – GPR125, UCHL1, THY1 and PLZF; RT-PCR for GPR123, GFRa1, RET, PLZF, UCHL1, MAGEA4, SYCP3, PRM1 and TNP1 at 30 d	22–35-year-old patients with obstructive azoospermia (n = 40)	Colonies of grapelike cells observed at 14 d, 1 mo, and 2 mo. Colonies stained for GPR125, THY1, UCHL1 and MAGEA4. No quantification.

Baert et al,[84] 2015	2 mo	Differential plating on plastic	StemPro-34	20 ng/mL EGF, 10 ng/mL GDNF, 10 ng/mL LIF, 10 ng/mL bFGF	No substrate	Not reported	ICC and RT-PCR - VASA, UCHL1	Vasectomy reversal patients and adult male patients who underwent bilateral orchidectomy due to prostate cancer (n = 6)	Single or small groups of VASA+/ UCHL1+ cells detected in considerable amounts up to 1 mo but infrequently after 2 mo.
Abdul Wahab et al,[97] 2016	49 d	Enrichment was not performed	DMEM	80 μl bFGF	Plastic	Not reported	In-well staining for ITGA6, ITGB1, CD9 and GFRA1	Non obstructive azoospermic male (n = 1)	Clusters observed until 49 d in culture. Some ITGA6+ and CD9+ cells were observed. No quantification.
Medrano et al,[96] 2016	28 d	FACS for HLA-/ EPCAM+	StemPro-34	20 ng/mL EGF, 10 ng/mL LIF, 10 ng/mL bFGF, 10 ng/mL GDNF	Testicular somatic cells	Not reported	ICC - Ki67; TUNEL; RT-PCR - UTF1, DAZL, VASA, PLZF, FGFR3, UCHL1; Elecsys Testosterone II competitive immunoassay; ELISA - Inhibin B	Adult male patients who underwent bilateral orchidectomy due to prostate cancer (n = 3)	VASA+/UTF1+ cells observed after 2 wk but were rarely Ki67+ and disappeared by 4 wk

(*continued on next page*)

Table 1
(continued)

Citation	Duration of Culture	Sort/ Differential Plating	Medium	Growth Factors	Feeders or ECM	Passaging Technique	End Point	Type and Age of Donor	Claim
Gat et al,[85] 2017	12 d	Differential plating on Gelatin	DMEM-F12 and StemPro-34	20 ng/mL EGF, 10 ng/mL GDNF, 10 ng/mL LIF, 10 ng/mL bFGF	Laminin and testicular somatic cells	Passaged using Trypsin when cells were 80%–90% confluent	SSC-like aggregates and targeted RNA seq for DAZL, ITGA6 and SYCP3	Adult orchidectomy patients (4 for testicular malignancies and 3 for testicular pain) and 1 adult who underwent microTESE due to NOA (n = 8)	Germ cell aggregates observed. Number impacted by medium and ratio of somatic cells to germ cells. No quantification over time.
Murdock et al,[93] 2018	14 d	MACS for ITGA6 followed by differential plating on Collagen I	MEMα	20 ng/mL GDNF, 1 ng/mL bFGF	STO, mouse and human laminin, htECM, ptECM, SIS, and UBM	Passaged using Trypsin at day 7	ICC – UTF1; flow cytometry – SSEA4, cKIT, AnnexinV and Ki-67	Adult organ donors (n = 4)	Aggregates observed. Number of UTF1+ cell declined over 14 d in culture.

Abbreviations: bFBF, basic fibroblast growth factor; DMEM, Dulbecco's modified Eagle's medium; ECM, extracellular matrix; EGF, epidermal growth factor; FACS, fluorescenceactivated cell sorting; FBS, fetal bovine serum; FCS, fetal calf serum; GDNF, glial cell line–derived neurotropic factor; htECM, human testis extracellular matrix; ITGA6, Integrin a6; ICC, immunocytochemistry; LIF, leukemia inhibitory factor; MACS, magnetic-activated cell sorting; MEM, minimum essential medium; MEF, mouse embryonic fibroblasts; NOA, nonobstructive azoospermia; PLZF, promyelocytic leukemia zinc finger; ptECM, porcine testis extracellular matrix; qPCR, quantitative polymerase chain reaction; qRT-PCR, quantitative reverse-transcriptase polymerase chain reaction; RBC, red blood cell; RT-PCR, reverse-transcriptase polymerase chain reaction; SIS, small intestine submucosa; SSC, spermatogonial stem cell; STO, SIM mouse embryonic fibroblasts; TGFB, transforming gorwoth factor beta; UBM, urinary bladder matrix.

Data from Refs.[18,77–97,112]

substrates that have been used for human SSC culture include human laminin, gelatin, Matrigel, Hydrogen Stem Easy, human and porcine testicular ECM, porcine small intestinal submucosa ECM, and urinary bladder ECM.[18,77,81,82,87,90,92,93] Most human SSC culture studies summarized in **Table 1** used culture conditions similar to what was originally described by Kanatsu-Shinohara and colleagues[71] in mouse and Sadri-Ardekani and colleagues[18] in human, including StemPro-34 medium supplemented with GDNF, basic fibroblast growth factor (bFGF), EGF, and LIF. Some of those studies reported significant expansion of spermatogonia in culture, suggesting an evolutionary conservation of factors required for SSC maintenance and proliferation,[18,77,90] although few studies have formally tested the requirement for those factors in human SSC culture.[78,80] Others reported a rapid decline in the number of human spermatogonia using those conditions.[83,84,91,96] The discrepancy in results can be explained in part by differences in starting cell populations and in part by different approaches to analysis of culture outcomes. Some studies reported the presence of clusters or colonies of putative spermatogonia with no attempt to quantify.[79,85,94] Some studies observed spermatogonial markers or xenotransplant colonizing activity in culture, but did not quantify.[78,81,86,88,89,92,95,97] Some quantified the number of clusters/colonies or total cells in culture but did not specifically quantify spermatogonia using markers or transplantation.[77,80,82,87,90] Finally, some studies quantified the number of cells with spermatogonial markers or xenotransplant colonizing activity over time in culture.[18,77,83,84,91,93,96]

CHALLENGES, OPPORTUNITIES, AND FUTURE DIRECTIONS

Variations in the methods for (1) selection of spermatogonia before culture, (2) culture conditions, and (3) analytical endpoints have made it difficult to compare studies or reach a consensus about optimal human SSC culture conditions. There are several cell surface markers that can be used to isolate and enrich human SSCs, but none of those can produce a pure population of SSCs. Therefore, any method used to sort before culture will produce a heterogeneous population of cells that is likely to include testicular germ cells and somatic cells. Quantification of colony or cluster number in culture is valuable but not sufficient as a single endpoint because it is possible to produce colonies of mesenchymal cells from human testes.[83,91]

Spermatogonial stem cell transplantation was the "gold-standard" assay that validated success expanding functional rodent SSCs in culture. Mouse and rat SSCs can colonize infertile mouse recipient testes and regenerate complete spermatogenesis.[28,29,98] Spermatogonial stem cell transplantation in humans is not possible as a routine biological assay, but human to nude mouse xenotransplantation has emerged as a powerful tool to quantify human spermatogonia with transplantation potential. Human cells do not produce complete spermatogenesis in mouse testes, but they do migrate to the basement membrane of seminiferous tubules, proliferate to produce characteristic chains and clusters of spermatogonia, and survive long-term.[64,99,100]

It is recognized that not all laboratories will have the expertise or infrastructure for human to nude mouse xenotransplantation. There has been significant progress in the last few years identifying protein markers of undifferentiated human stem/progenitor spermatogonia (eg, UTF1, PIWIL4, UCHL1, PLZF, SALL4, GFRA1, LPPR3, TCF3, TSPAN33, and others).[100–103] These markers can be detected and quantified at a single-cell level using immunocytochemistry or flow cytometry. Reverse-transcriptase PCR (RT-PCR) is a complementary and sensitive method to confirm the presence of spermatogonial transcripts but does not reveal protein expression or provide information about spermatogonial quantity. Similarly, markers that are expressed by spermatogonia and other somatic cell types in the testis can be misleading (eg, ITGA6, THY1, UCHL1).[84,91,95,96] Multiparameter staining (eg, VASA+/UCHL1+) may help to resolve these issues.[84,96] Spermatogonial marker–positive cells should be monitored and quantified throughout the culture period and not just the end because this will help to understand spermatogonial proliferation dynamics over time. Complementing markers of undifferentiated spermatogonia with markers of differentiation (eg, cKIT), apoptosis (eg, annexinV, Caspase 3), and proliferation (eg, ki67) will help elucidate the fate of spermatogonia once they are placed in culture.

The growth requirements to maintain or expand human SSCs in culture are not known. Many studies have started with factors that were used in mouse SSC culture (any combination of GDNF, bFGF, EGF, and LIF), but few have formally tested the requirement for those factors.[78,80] Characterization of human germ and testicular somatic cells through single-cell RNA sequencing may help shed light on additional factors or signaling pathways in human SSCs that might be manipulated in culture to promote SSC survival and/or proliferation or new markers that can be used to isolate and enrich human SSCs.[101,102,104]

Mouse and rat SSCs divide once every 3 to 11 days in culture, similar to their in vivo proliferation dynamics. The in vivo cell cycle time of undifferentiated human A_{dark} and A_{pale} spermatogonia ranges from 1.5 to 8.0 months. If, like rodents, human SSC proliferation dynamics in culture are similar to the in vivo situation, it raises questions about whether it will ever be possible to expand human SSC numbers in culture. An emerging alternative approach could be to expand patient-derived induced pluripotent stem cells (iPSCs) in culture and then differentiate them into primordial germ cell–like cells (PGCLCs).[105–109] PGCLCs can potentially be transplanted into the testes to regenerate spermatogenesis[110] or differentiated to sperm in vitro,[111] outcomes that have been reported in mice, but not yet for any other species.

Despite the challenges outlined in this article, culture of human male germline stem cells, including SSCs or iPSC-derived PGCLCs, will have important applications for fundamental investigations of human germ lineage development and spermatogenesis. This is important because our current understanding of human SSC function and spermatogenesis is based primarily on data generated in mice. Knowledge generated from human germline stem cell culture could have important implications for development of next-generation reproductive technologies using stem cells.

ACKNOWLEDGMENTS

KEO is supported by donor funds administered by Magee-Womens Research Institute and Foundation and by NIH grants HD075795; HD082084; HD076412; HD096723.

REFERENCES

1. Siegel RL, Miller KD, Jemal A. Cancer statistics, 2018. CA Cancer J Clin 2018;68(1):7–30.
2. Jacobsen PB, Jim HSL. Consideration of quality of life in cancer survivorship research. Cancer Epidemiol Biomarkers Prev 2011;20(10):2035–41.
3. Hammond C, Abrams JR, Syrjala KL. Fertility and risk factors for elevated infertility concern in 10-year hematopoietic cell transplant survivors and case-matched controls. J Clin Oncol 2007;25(23):3511–7.
4. Howell SJ, Shalet SM. Spermatogenesis after cancer treatment: damage and recovery. J Natl Cancer Inst Monogr 2005;2005(34):12–7.
5. Okada K, Fujisawa M. Recovery of spermatogenesis following cancer treatment with cytotoxic chemotherapy and radiotherapy. World J Mens Health 2019;37(2):166–74.
6. Agarwal A, Ong C, Durairajanayagam D. Contemporary and future insights into fertility preservation in male cancer patients. Transl Androl Urol 2014; 3(1):27–40.
7. Wallace WH, Anderson RA, Irvine DS. Fertility preservation for young patients with cancer: who is at risk and what can be offered? Lancet Oncol 2005;6(4):209–18.
8. Green DM, Nolan VG, Goodman PJ, et al. The cyclophosphamide equivalent dose as an approach for quantifying alkylating agent exposure: a report from the Childhood Cancer Survivor Study. Pediatr Blood Cancer 2014;61(1):53–67.
9. Su IH, Lee YT, Barr R. Oncofertility: meeting the fertility goals of adolescents and young adults with cancer. Cancer J 2018;24(6):328–35.
10. Loren AW, Mangu PB, Beck LN, et al. Fertility preservation for patients with cancer: American Society of Clinical Oncology clinical practice guideline update. J Clin Oncol 2013;31(19):2500–10.
11. Fallat ME, Hutter J. Preservation of fertility in pediatric and adolescent patients with cancer. Pediatrics 2008;121(5):e1461–9.
12. Practice Committee of American Society for Reproductive Medicine. Fertility preservation in patients undergoing gonadotoxic therapy or gonadectomy: a committee opinion. Fertil Sterility 2019;112(6):1022–33.
13. Oktay K, Harvey BE, Partridge AH, et al. Fertility preservation in patients with cancer: ASCO clinical practice guideline update. J Clin Oncol 2018; 36(19):1994–2001.
14. Shankara-Narayana N, Di Pierro I, Fennell C, et al. Sperm cryopreservation prior to gonadotoxic treatment: experience of a single academic centre over 4 decades. Hum Reprod 2019;34(5):795–803.
15. Fu L, Zhou F, An Q, et al. Sperm cryopreservation for male cancer patients: more than 10 years of experience, in Beijing China. Med Sci Monit 2019; 25:3256–61.
16. Bahadur G, Chatterjee R, Ralph D. Testicular tissue cryopreservation in boys. Ethical and legal issues: case report. Hum Reprod 2000;15(6):1416–20.
17. Keros V, Hultenby K, Borgstrom B, et al. Methods of cryopreservation of testicular tissue with viable spermatogonia in pre-pubertal boys undergoing gonadotoxic cancer treatment. Hum Reprod 2007;22(5):1384–95.
18. Sadri-Ardekani H, Mizrak SC, van Daalen SK, et al. Propagation of human spermatogonial stem cells in vitro. JAMA 2009;302(19):2127–34.
19. Ginsberg JP. New advances in fertility preservation for pediatric cancer patients. Curr Opin Pediatr 2011;23(1):9–13.
20. Wyns C, Curaba M, Petit S, et al. Management of fertility preservation in prepubertal patients: 5 years' experience at the Catholic University of Louvain. Hum Reprod 2011;26(4):737–47.
21. Pietzak EJ Iii, Tasian GE, Tasian SK, et al. Histology of testicular biopsies obtained for experimental

fertility preservation protocol in boys with cancer. J Urol 2015;194(5):1420–4.
22. Stukenborg JB, Alves-Lopes JP, Kurek M, et al. Spermatogonial quantity in human prepubertal testicular tissue collected for fertility preservation prior to potentially sterilizing therapy. Hum Reprod 2018;33:1677–83.
23. Valli-Pulaski H, Peters KA, Gassei K, et al. Testicular tissue cryopreservation: 8 years of experience from a coordinated network of academic centers. Hum Reprod 2019;34(6):966–77.
24. Gassei K, Orwig KE. Experimental methods to preserve male fertility and treat male factor infertility. Fertil Steril 2016;105(2):256–66.
25. Medrano JV, Andres MDM, Garcia S, et al. Basic and clinical approaches for fertility preservation and restoration in cancer patients. Trends Biotechnol 2018;36(2):199–215.
26. Radford JA, Shalet SM, Lieberman BA. Fertility after treatment for cancer. BMJ 1999;319(7215): 935–6.
27. Radford J. Restoration of fertility after treatment for cancer. Horm Res 2003;59(Suppl 1):21–3.
28. Brinster RL, Avarbock MR. Germline transmission of donor haplotype following spermatogonial transplantation. Proc Natl Acad Sci U S A 1994;91(24): 11303–7.
29. Brinster RL, Zimmermann JW. Spermatogenesis following male germ-cell transplantation. Proc Natl Acad Sci U S A 1994;91(24):11298–302.
30. Honaramooz A, Behboodi E, Megee SO, et al. Fertility and germline transmission of donor haplotype following germ cell transplantation in immunocompetent goats. Biol Reprod 2003;69(4):1260–4.
31. Kim Y, Turner D, Nelson J, et al. Production of donor-derived sperm after spermatogonial stem cell transplantation in the dog. Reproduction 2008;136(6):823–31.
32. Herrid M, Olejnik J, Jackson M, et al. Irradiation enhances the efficiency of testicular germ cell transplantation in sheep. Biol Reprod 2009;81(5): 898–905.
33. Hermann BP, Sukhwani M, Winkler F, et al. Spermatogonial stem cell transplantation into rhesus testes regenerates spermatogenesis producing functional sperm. Cell Stem Cell 2012;11(5): 715–26.
34. Izadyar F, Den Ouden K, Stout TA, et al. Autologous and homologous transplantation of bovine spermatogonial stem cells. Reproduction 2003;126(6): 765–74.
35. Schlatt S, Foppiani L, Rolf C, et al. Germ cell transplantation into X-irradiated monkey testes. Hum Reprod 2002;17(1):55–62.
36. Mikkola M, Sironen A, Kopp C, et al. Transplantation of normal boar testicular cells resulted in complete focal spermatogenesis in a boar affected by the immotile short-tail sperm defect. Reprod Domest Anim 2006;41(2):124–8.
37. Shinohara T, Orwig KE, Avarbock MR, et al. Remodeling of the postnatal mouse testis is accompanied by dramatic changes in stem cell number and niche accessibility. Proc Natl Acad Sci U S A 2001;98(11):6186–91.
38. Ryu BY, Orwig KE, Avarbock MR, et al. Stem cell and niche development in the postnatal rat testis. Developmental Biol 2003;263(2):253–63.
39. Dobrinski I, Avarbock MR, Brinster RL. Transplantation of germ cells from rabbits and dogs into mouse testes. Biol Reprod 1999;61(5):1331–9.
40. Dobrinski I, Avarbock MR, Brinster RL. Germ cell transplantation from large domestic animals into mouse testes. Mol Reprod Dev 2000;57(3):270–9.
41. Wu X, Goodyear SM, Abramowitz LK, et al. Fertile offspring derived from mouse spermatogonial stem cells cryopreserved for more than 14 years. Hum Reprod 2012;27(5):1249–59.
42. Ogawa T, Arechaga JM, Avarbock MR, et al. Transplantation of testis germinal cells into mouse seminiferous tubules. Int J Dev Biol 1997;41(1): 111–22.
43. Schlatt S, Rosiepen G, Weinbauer GF, et al. Germ cell transfer into rat, bovine, monkey and human testes. Hum Reprod 1999;14(1):144–50.
44. Honaramooz A, Megee SO, Dobrinski I. Germ cell transplantation in pigs. Biol Reprod 2002;66(1): 21–8.
45. Kanatsu-Shinohara M, Takehashi M, Takashima S, et al. Homing of mouse spermatogonial stem cells to germline niche depends on beta1-integrin. Cell Stem Cell 2008;3(5):533–42.
46. Takashima S, Kanatsu-Shinohara M, Tanaka T, et al. Rac mediates mouse spermatogonial stem cell homing to germline niches by regulating transmigration through the blood-testis barrier. Cell Stem Cell 2011;9(5):463–75.
47. Parreira GG, Ogawa T, Avarbock MR, et al. Development of germ cell transplants in mice. Biol Reprod 1998;59(6):1360–70.
48. Nagano M, Avarbock MR, Brinster RL. Pattern and kinetics of mouse donor spermatogonial stem cell colonization in recipient testes. Biol Reprod 1999; 60(6):1429–36.
49. Braye A, Tournaye H, Goossens E. Setting up a cryopreservation programme for immature testicular tissue: lessons learned after more than 15 years of experience. Clin Med Insights Reprod Health 2019;13. 1179558119886342.
50. Seandel M, James D, Shmelkov SV, et al. Generation of functional multipotent adult stem cells from GPR125+ germline progenitors. Nature 2007; 449(7160):346–50.
51. Shinohara T, Avarbock MR, Brinster RL. beta1- and alpha6-integrin are surface markers on mouse

spermatogonial stem cells. Proc Natl Acad Sci U S A 1999;96(10):5504–9.
52. Kanatsu-Shinohara M, Toyokuni S, Shinohara T. CD9 is a surface marker on mouse and rat male germline stem cells. Biol Reprod 2004;70(1):70–5.
53. Kubota H, Avarbock MR, Brinster RL. Spermatogonial stem cells share some, but not all, phenotypic and functional characteristics with other stem cells. Proc Natl Acad Sci U S A 2003;100(11):6487–92.
54. Tadokoro Y, Yomogida K, Ohta H, et al. Homeostatic regulation of germinal stem cell proliferation by the GDNF/FSH pathway. Mech Dev 2002;113(1):29–39.
55. Garbuzov A, Pech MF, Hasegawa K, et al. Purification of GFRα1+ and GFRα1– spermatogonial stem cells reveals a niche-dependent mechanism for fate determination. Stem Cell Reports 2018;10(2):553–67.
56. Kubota H, Avarbock MR, Schmidt JA, et al. Spermatogonial stem cells derived from infertile Wv/Wv mice self-renew in vitro and generate progeny following transplantation. Biol Reprod 2009;81(2):293–301.
57. Shinohara T, Orwig KE, Avarbock MR, et al. Spermatogonial stem cell enrichment by multiparameter selection of mouse testis cells. Proc Natl Acad Sci U S A 2000;97(15):8346–51.
58. Fujita K, Ohta H, Tsujimura A, et al. Transplantation of spermatogonial stem cells isolated from leukemic mice restores fertility without inducing leukemia. J Clin Invest 2005;115(7):1855–61.
59. von Kopylow K, Kirchhoff C, Jezek D, et al. Screening for biomarkers of spermatogonia within the human testis: a whole genome approach. Hum Reprod 2010;25(5):1104–12.
60. Izadyar F, Wong J, Maki C, et al. Identification and characterization of repopulating spermatogonial stem cells from the adult human testis. Hum Reprod 2011;26(6):1296–306.
61. Guo J, Grow EJ, Mlcochova H, et al. The adult human testis transcriptional cell atlas. Cell Res 2018;28(12):1141–57.
62. Jahnukainen K, Hou M, Petersen C, et al. Intratesticular transplantation of testicular cells from leukemic rats causes transmission of leukemia. Cancer Res 2001;61(2):706–10.
63. Fujita K, Tsujimura A, Miyagawa Y, et al. Isolation of germ cells from leukemia and lymphoma cells in a human in vitro model: potential clinical application for restoring human fertility after anticancer therapy. Cancer Res 2006;66(23):11166–71.
64. Dovey SL, Valli H, Hermann BP, et al. Eliminating malignant contamination from therapeutic human spermatogonial stem cells. J Clin Invest 2013;123(4):1833–43.
65. Hermann BP, Sukhwani M, Salati J, et al. Separating spermatogonia from cancer cells in contaminated prepubertal primate testis cell suspensions. Hum Reprod 2011;26(12):3222–31.
66. Geens M, Van de Velde H, De Block G, et al. The efficiency of magnetic-activated cell sorting and fluorescence-activated cell sorting in the decontamination of testicular cell suspensions in cancer patients. Hum Reprod 2007;22(3):733–42.
67. Courbiere B, Prebet T, Mozziconacci MJ, et al. Tumor cell contamination in ovarian tissue cryopreserved before gonadotoxic treatment: should we systematically exclude ovarian autograft in a cancer survivor? Bone Marrow Transplant 2010;45(7):1247–8.
68. Dolmans MM, Marinescu C, Saussoy P, et al. Reimplantation of cryopreserved ovarian tissue from patients with acute lymphoblastic leukemia is potentially unsafe. Blood 2010;116(16):2908–14.
69. Sadri-Ardekani H, Atala A. Testicular tissue cryopreservation and spermatogonial stem cell transplantation to restore fertility: from bench to bedside. Stem Cell Res Ther 2014;5(3):68.
70. Meng X, Lindahl M, Hyvonen ME, et al. Regulation of cell fate decision of undifferentiated spermatogonia by GDNF. Science 2000;287(5457):1489–93.
71. Kanatsu-Shinohara M, Ogonuki N, Inoue K, et al. Long-term proliferation in culture and germline transmission of mouse male germline stem cells. Biol Reprod 2003;69(2):612–6.
72. Kubota H, Avarbock MR, Brinster RL. Culture conditions and single growth factors affect fate determination of mouse spermatogonial stem cells. Biol Reprod 2004;71(3):722–31.
73. Kubota H, Avarbock MR, Brinster RL. Growth factors essential for self-renewal and expansion of mouse spermatogonial stem cells. Proc Natl Acad Sci U S A 2004;101(47):16489–94.
74. Oatley JM, Avarbock MR, Brinster RL. Glial cell line-derived neurotrophic factor regulation of genes essential for self-renewal of mouse spermatogonial stem cells is dependent on Src family kinase signaling. J Biol Chem 2007;282(35):25842–51.
75. Hamra FK, Chapman KM, Nguyen DM, et al. Self renewal, expansion, and transfection of rat spermatogonial stem cells in culture. Proc Natl Acad Sci U S A 2005;102(48):17430–5.
76. Ryu BY, Kubota H, Avarbock MR, et al. Conservation of spermatogonial stem cell self-renewal signaling between mouse and rat. Proc Natl Acad Sci U S A 2005;102(40):14302–7.
77. Sadri-Ardekani H, Akhondi MA, van der Veen F, et al. In vitro propagation of human prepubertal spermatogonial stem cells. JAMA 2011;305(23):2416–8.
78. Wu X, Schmidt JA, Avarbock MR, et al. Prepubertal human spermatogonia and mouse gonocytes share conserved gene expression of germline

stem cell regulatory molecules. Proc Natl Acad Sci U S A 2009;106(51):21672–7.
79. Nowroozi MR, Ahmadi H, Rafiian S, et al. In vitro colonization of human spermatogonia stem cells: effect of patient's clinical characteristics and testicular histologic findings. Urology 2011;78(5): 1075–81.
80. Mirzapour T, Movahedin M, Tengku Ibrahim TA, et al. Effects of basic fibroblast growth factor and leukaemia inhibitory factor on proliferation and short-term culture of human spermatogonial stem cells. Andrologia 2012;44:41–55.
81. Goharbakhsh L, Mohazzab A, Salehkhou S, et al. Isolation and culture of human spermatogonial stem cells derived from testis biopsy. Avicenna J Med Biotechnol 2013;5(1):54–61.
82. Piravar Z, Jeddi-Tehrani M, Sadeghi MR, et al. In vitro culture of human testicular stem cells on feeder-free condition. J Reprod Infertil 2013;14(1): 17–22.
83. Zheng Y, Thomas A, Schmidt CM, et al. Quantitative detection of human spermatogonia for optimization of spermatogonial stem cell culture. Hum Reprod 2014;29(11):2497–511.
84. Baert Y, Braye A, Struijk RB, et al. Cryopreservation of testicular tissue before long-term testicular cell culture does not alter in vitro cell dynamics. Fertil Steril 2015;104(5):1244–52.e1-4.
85. Gat I, Maghen L, Filice M, et al. Optimal culture conditions are critical for efficient expansion of human testicular somatic and germ cells in vitro. Fertil Sterility 2017;107(3):595–605.e7.
86. Koruji M, Shahverdi A, Janan A, et al. Proliferation of small number of human spermatogonial stem cells obtained from azoospermic patients. J Assist Reprod Genet 2012;29(9):957–67.
87. Lim JJ, Sung SY, Kim HJ, et al. Long-term proliferation and characterization of human spermatogonial stem cells obtained from obstructive and non-obstructive azoospermia under exogenous feeder-free culture conditions. Cell Prolif 2010; 43(4):405–17.
88. Liu S, Tang Z, Xiong T, et al. Isolation and characterization of human spermatogonial stem cells. Reprod Biol Endocrinol 2011;9:141.
89. He ZP, Kokkinaki M, Jiang JJ, et al. Isolation, characterization, and culture of human spermatogonia. Biol Reprod 2010;82(2):363–72.
90. Kokkinaki M, Djourabtchi A, Golestaneh N. Long-term culture of human SSEA-4 positive spermatogonial stem cells (SSCs). J Stem Cell Res Ther 2011;S2:003.
91. Chikhovskaya JV, van Daalen SKM, Korver CM, et al. Mesenchymal origin of multipotent human testis-derived stem cells in human testicular cell cultures. Mol Hum Reprod 2014;20(2):155–67.
92. Guo Y, Liu L, Sun M, et al. Expansion and long-term culture of human spermatogonial stem cells via the activation of SMAD3 and AKT pathways. Exp Biol Med (Maywood) 2015;240(8):1112–22.
93. Murdock MH, David S, Swinehart IT, et al. Human testis extracellular matrix enhances human spermatogonial stem cell survival in vitro. Tissue Eng Part A 2019;25(7–8):663–76.
94. Chen B, Wang YB, Zhang ZL, et al. Xeno-free culture of human spermatogonial stem cells supported by human embryonic stem cell-derived fibroblast-like cells. Asian J Androl 2009;11(5): 557–65.
95. Smith JF, Yango P, Altman E, et al. Testicular niche required for human spermatogonial stem cell expansion. Stem Cell Transl Med 2014;3(9): 1043–54.
96. Medrano JV, Rombaut C, Simon C, et al. Human spermatogonial stem cells display limited proliferation in vitro under mouse spermatogonial stem cell culture conditions. Fertil Steril 2016;106(6): 1539–49.e8.
97. Abdul Wahab AY, Md Isa ML, Ramli R. Spermatogonial stem cells protein identification in in vitro culture from non-obstructive azoospermia patient. Malays J Med Sci 2016;23(3):40–8.
98. Clouthier DE, Avarbock MR, Maika SD, et al. Rat spermatogenesis in mouse testis. Nature 1996; 381(6581):418–21.
99. Nagano M, Patrizio P, Brinster RL. Long-term survival of human spermatogonial stem cells in mouse testes. Fertil Steril 2002;78(6):1225–33.
100. Valli H, Sukhwani M, Dovey SL, et al. Fluorescence- and magnetic-activated cell sorting strategies to isolate and enrich human spermatogonial stem cells. Fertil Steril 2014;102(2):566–80.
101. Guo J, Grow EJ, Yi C, et al. Chromatin and single-cell RNA-Seq profiling reveal dynamic signaling and metabolic transitions during human spermatogonial stem cell development. Cell Stem Cell 2017; 21(4):533–46.e6.
102. Sohni A, Tan K, Song HW, et al. The neonatal and adult human testis defined at the single-cell level. Cell Rep 2019;26(6):1501–17.e4.
103. von Kopylow K, Spiess AN. Human spermatogonial markers. Stem Cell Res 2017;25:300–9.
104. Hermann BP, Cheng K, Singh A, et al. The mammalian spermatogenesis single-cell transcriptome, from spermatogonial stem cells to spermatids. Cell Rep 2018;25(6):1650–67.e8.
105. Clark AT, Bodnar MS, Fox M, et al. Spontaneous differentiation of germ cells from human embryonic stem cells in vitro. Hum Mol Genet 2004;13(7): 727–39.
106. Durruthy Durruthy J, Ramathal C, Sukhwani M, et al. Fate of induced pluripotent stem cells

following transplantation to murine seminiferous tubules. Hum Mol Genet 2014;23(12):3071–84.

107. Park TS, Galic Z, Conway AE, et al. Derivation of primordial germ cells from human embryonic and induced pluripotent stem cells is significantly improved by coculture with human fetal gonadal cells. Stem Cells 2009;27(4):783–95.

108. Chen D, Liu W, Zimmerman J, et al. The TFAP2C-regulated OCT4 naive enhancer is involved in human germline formation. Cell Rep 2018;25(13):3591–602.e5.

109. Irie N, Surani MA. Efficient induction and isolation of human primordial germ cell-like cells from competent human pluripotent stem cells. Methods Mol Biol 2017;1463:217–26.

110. Hayashi K, Ohta H, Kurimoto K, et al. Reconstitution of the mouse germ cell specification pathway in culture by pluripotent stem cells. Cell 2011;146(4):519–32.

111. Zhou Q, Wang M, Yuan Y, et al. Complete meiosis from embryonic stem cell-derived germ cells in vitro. Cell Stem Cell 2016;18(3):330–40.

112. Akhondi MM, Mohazzab A, Jeddi-Tehrani M, et al. Propagation of human germ stem cells in long-term culture. Iran J Reprod Med 2013;11(7):551–8.

Personalized Medicine in Infertile Men

Nicolás Garrido, PhD, MSc*, Irene Hervás, MSc

KEYWORDS

• Male infertility • Personalized medicine • Sperm • Molecular biomarkers • OMICS

KEY POINTS

- Male infertility is a heterogeneous disorder that is responsible for 30% of cases of infertility in the couple. Occasionally, its diagnose remain incomplete or unknown.
- Personalized medicine is a new approach in clinical assistance, providing a prevention, diagnose and treatment tailored for each patient.
- The omics technologies enhance the knowledge in the human reproduction field, permitting a deeper insight of male gamete and the molecular origin of infertility.
- The identification of novel molecules involved in sperm function and used them as biomarkers may provide a new diagnostic tool and the improvement of sperm selection techniques.
- Personalized medicine promises to be a both diagnostic and therapeutic tool in the clinic management of male infertility, providing a new medical approach toward individualization of infertility treatment.

WHAT IS PERSONALIZED MEDICINE?

Personalized medicine can be defined as the application of specific medical techniques, drugs and/or processes to individual patients to prevent, diagnose, or cure disease, in contrast with the old approach of treating them all similarly, based on the detailed knowledge of unique and explicit characteristics of the individual's and the disease, at either the genotype, physiology, environmental exposure, or lifestyle, among other factors, levels in a precise and tailor-made form. It is a revolutionary approach for disease prevention and treatment that considers individual variability into all areas of health care.[1] To this end, knowing the exact causes of the disease, and the underlying physiology, is key when trying to develop tools to treat, and from this approach, more effectively, efficiently, and with fewer side effects, are expected thus resulting in a benefit for all patients.

Similarly, this term is often also designated as precision medicine, aiming, for instance, to stratify diseases, patients, or responses to drugs in taxonomic groups, and to predict more accurately which treatment and prevention strategies for particular disorders will be efficient in homogeneous groups of people.[2,3] It is a change compared with the traditional one-size-fits-all approach, in which both the disease prevention and treatment are designed for the average person or population. This new strategy makes medicine personalized, preventive, predictive, and participatory for each patient.[3]

These concepts were born at the beginning of the 21st century, just after the publication of the Human Genome Project in 2003.[4] Thanks to this revolutionary milestone, the way of understanding the diagnosis and treatment of human diseases has evolved from generality to individuality, and such transformation has been possible owing, among other factors, to the development in

Fundación Instituto Valenciano de Infertilidad (FIVI), Instituto Universitario IVI (IUIVI), Avda. Fernando Abril Martorell, no106, Torre A, Planta 1ª, Valencia 46026, Spain
* Corresponding author.
E-mail address: nicolas.garrido@ivirma.com

Urol Clin N Am 47 (2020) 245–255
https://doi.org/10.1016/j.ucl.2019.12.011

parallel of high-output molecular analyses techniques and computational tools based on big data and large-scale data management, for instance, from the different -omic sciences.[5,6] All these developments permitted imagining a new approach, unthinkable just decades before.

This change in health management includes a deeper comprehension about individual's information to determine predisposition to specific diseases and to predict the efficacy or safety of treatments, as well as opening the possibility to develop patient-specific treating approaches. The aim is to provide personalized assistance in[7]:

- Prevention: analysis of (among other factors) genomic information to know the individual susceptibility to develop a disease, allowing its early detection rather than their observing later clinical manifestations, and also, to improve the ability to predict which treatment will work best in each case, to increase efficiency.[6,8]
- Diagnosis: understanding of the origin, underlying risk factors, molecular mechanisms involved, and genetic variants responsible of the occurrence of the disease to develop and use specific biomarkers to detect, classify, and monitor the course of disease.[2,9,10]
- Treatment: establish a specific therapy based on the disease's intrinsic and specific features[5] and tailored to the patient, considering the genetic, biochemical, physiologic and environmental patient's traits.[1,2]

To date, as an example, there are approaches to personalized medicine at different levels, in medical specialties such as oncology and immunology, where the approach to the problem goes from the study of the genetic profile of the patient and the disease (as in the case of tumors), to some cases where a personalized medical treatment can be established and adjusted to increase the effectiveness and possibilities of recovery, against what the historical method to solve the health problem has been.[1,11]

The wider application of such methods in other medicine fields is expected to be introduced sooner than later, and the current trend from general to more specific, and even personalized approaches, in preventing, diagnosing, and treating are now, to some extent, often present when dealing with infertile patients, including infertile males.

WHAT IS KNOWN ABOUT MALE INFERTILITY, WHAT REMAINS TO BE DEFINED, AND HOW CLOSE ARE WE TO THE PERSONALIZED MEDICINE IN MALE INFERTILITY

The social impact of infertility can be considered high, because nearly 15% of couples at their reproductive ages are unable to conceive after 1 year of unprotected intercourse.[12] According to the American Society for Reproductive Medicine, male factor infertility is responsible for 30% of cases of infertility in the couple and roughly speaking 40% can be attributed to female causes. The remaining 30% is usually classified as caused by the combination of both female and male factors, or simply remains unexplained so far (the so-called idiopathic infertility).[13,14]

Male infertility, considered as the inability of a male to satisfy his reproductive aims through sexual intercourse, can be considered as a multifactorial disorder, in some cases caused by known and specific causes such as chromosomal abnormalities, infections, gene mutations, varicocele, hormonal disruption, or reproductive tract obstructions, among others,[15] that result in the impossibility or reduction of the conceiving likelihood. These causes can be temporary or permanent, and can also be divided between men able to produce low numbers and/or physiologically incompetent spermatozoa, or those unable to complete spermatogenesis.

From this variety of possibilities, it seems obvious that there is a need to approach each case individually.

Currently, the routine evaluation of male infertility is mainly based on semen analysis. This technique evaluates semen quality by means of measuring the ejaculate macro and microscopic parameters as sperm cell density, motility, morphology and viability, according to World Health Organization's manual criteria.[16]

However, it does not provide predictive information on the fertile potential in males, nor for fertilization or the assisted reproduction treatment success.[17] A normal result of semen analysis does not guarantee fertility and none of the semen parameters indicate a proper sperm physiologic function. In fact, 30% of normozoospermic men are unable to achieve pregnancy.[18] This limitation as a predictive test does not imply that basic semen analysis results are not a cost-effective way to estimate fertility potential, decide which are the most convenient therapeutic approaches and assisted reproduction techniques to be used, and also detect cases where additional tests may be required to better discern the causes of infertility and/or avoid reproductive risks to the offspring.

Facing that situation, a more detailed physical and clinical examination should be performed.[19] For instance, the absence of spermatozoa or the presence of abnormal sperm in the ejaculate may reflect chromosomic disorders. Nowadays, to investigate the genetic origin of a disrupted spermatogenesis, the clinically relevant test are karyotype and Y-linked microdeletions assays.[15]

The karyotype is one of the genetic tests used to complement male infertility evaluation where the sperm counts are low and permits the chromosome structure to be examined. The karyotype anomalies are related to chromosomic deletions or translocations, that, ultimately, affect sperm production,[20,21] showing reduction in sperm concentration.

In contrast, the study of the microdeletions of the Y-chromosome is performed to inspect the chromosome integrity. These microdeletions affect azoospermia factor genes and it is associated with severe oligospermic and azoospermic men. Clinical evaluation of Y-chromosome microdeletions may the opportunity to find sperm in a testicular biopsy,[15,22] and also the possibility to transmit this condition to the progeny. Genetic counseling is needed in these cases.[22]

This clinical evaluation of male infertility is to some extent superficial and limited, and does not examine the concomitant sperm physiology related to fertility. Spermatozoa can be considered as the most specialized cells within the human body. The male gamete is more than the carrier of genetic information from the progenitor, because it provides, among other things, proteins and RNA-rich cytoplasm to the future embryo,[23,24] that are well-related with reproductive success.

The spermatogenesis is a complex and highly specific process that requires an exact coordination of the molecular pathways involved.[25] A failure in these processes involves the formation of immature and/or dysfunctional sperm cells. If the sperm's competence to trigger a correct embryonic development is compromised, it will be reflected in poor results in assisted reproduction cycles.

The molecular factors related to fertilization failures, poor embryonic quality, or poor clinical outcomes cannot be completely explained with conventional semen analyses so far. Besides, there are other sperm intrinsic characteristics impossible to be assessed only by means of spermiogram requiring other specific tests.[26] Within such characteristics, one may find DNA fragmentation, chromatin compaction, membrane integrity, and maturity or apoptosis level,[23,26] and also a significant number of investigational tests not translated yet to the clinical practice, but pretending to satisfy a personalized medicine approach. This fact clearly denotes the need to develop new male infertility tests. The improvements required are closely link with the need to find and to select the best quality sperm before attempting in vitro fertilization or intracytoplasmic sperm injection (ICSI)[27] to achieve an ongoing pregnancy and a healthy infant, or enabling the selection of one specific sperm sample among several ejaculates from the same male because of their specific probabilities of success. Sperm selection techniques based on molecular traits are going to be one of the strategies designed with this purpose. The objective of these methods is to isolate sperm with the best characteristics from the seminal sample to fertilize the oocytes,[28] mimicking the natural selection process realized by the female reproductive tract.[23]

Broadly, these techniques select or deselect sperm based on their molecular characteristics, such as apoptosis markers (like in magnetic activated cell sorting), sperm surface charge, or its ability to bind to hyaluronic acid (physiologic intracytoplasmic sperm injection). In contrast, other selection techniques assess the male gamete morphology at higher magnification (intracytoplasmic morphologically selected sperm injection) or its birefringence.[23,27,28]

With these techniques, the sperm cell is not damaged, nor is integrity endangered, and after isolating them, the spermatozoa can be used for reproduction purposes coupled with assisted reproduction techniques afterward. Currently, some of the molecules linked to fertility in sperm, where a specific sperm selection methodology has been developed and are currently available to select sperm are phosphatidyl serine (apoptosis marker), ubiquitin (defective sperm marker), and phospholipase A2 (sperm capacitation).[23] Conversely, negative selection isolates a sperm pool with inadequate molecular characteristics, discarding them, and enriching in physiologically better spermatozoa, ultimately obtaining a seminal sample enriched with the most competent cells is obtained, aiming to improve the success of assisted reproduction treatments.[29]

Nevertheless, despite the theoretic benefit of these selection methods, the latest reviews noted that clinical outcomes (implantation, pregnancy, and live birth rates) cannot be enhanced by means of current sperm selection techniques,[27,28] or in other cases, clinical information is still lacking. At present, regardless of an active effort to identify the causes of male infertility, a lot of men are undiagnosed and other are unable to have offspring without a justified reason.

New diagnostic techniques are necessary to ascertain the cause of infertility and to recognize both semen and sperm quality, and to design appropriate strategies for fertility treatment or sperm selection, optimizing clinical outcomes.[23] In this respect, personalized medicine is a new approach in the diagnosis of male infertility and its clinical treatment.

PERSONALIZED REPRODUCTIVE MEDICINE

Personalized medicine approaches have a great potential as diagnostic and therapeutic tool in the field of human reproduction and infertility treatment. Knowing the different molecular and pathophysiologic mechanisms that result in infertility is one of the focal points from which to establish an appropriate diagnosis and treatment for each couple.

Individual differences in disease development and in response to medication as a result of genetic and environment differences are evident. Therefore, the classical one-size-fits-all approach in infertility treatments does no benefit everyone and should be abandoned. The focus of assisted reproduction techniques should to evolve toward individualization of infertility treatment, tailoring the treatment according to the patient's conditions and requirements, with the aim to increase the chance of achieving a live birth. In this sense, personalized reproductive medicine is a good opportunity to improve the efficiency of assisted reproduction treatments and their cost effectiveness, decreasing both the number of cycles needed and the cost of treatment, as well as diminishing the patient's emotional burden.[30]

This approach has already been applied in the management of female infertility. Treatment individualization is carried out in ovarian stimulation protocols, tailored to their own prediction of ovarian response. For instance, the anti-Mullerian hormone value and the antral follicle count determine the dosses necessary for ovarian stimulation, avoiding both a poor or hyper response.[31] Another example is embryo transfer according to the receptivity stage of endometrium (window of implantation), which differs between patients.[32] This strategy maximizes the chances of implantation in cases where the patient shows a displacement on the receptive period, and consequently, pregnancy likelihood.

Nonetheless, male infertility remains partly unexplored, and greater effort is needed to optimize diagnosis and treatment. Owing to the limitations presented by semen analysis as a diagnostic (and predictive) tool, new effective methods should be created for the establishment of the infertility etiology, identification of fertilization potential, and prediction of the most efficacy therapy.

Personalized medicine can largely benefit male's reproductive health by helping to prevent, diagnose and treat diseases related to the male reproductive system.[33] For example, understanding how genes are associated with certain disease onset has been helpful in, for example, prostate cancer and benign prostatic hyperplasia.

Patients who carry a mutation may know the susceptibility to develop a specific disease; being a BRCA1/2 or HOXB13 gene mutation carrier increases prostate cancer risk, but also allows for the planning of an appropriate prevention program. In patients with benign prostatic hyperplasia, different single nucleotide polymorphism variants are associated with different degrees of disease aggressiveness. In both cases, its understanding led to the development of targeted pharmacogenomic therapies that improve healing.[34]

Personalized medicine in male infertility management seems promising. Technological advances have unraveled a myriad of molecular factors involved in reproduction function and, thus, sperm physiology.

The emergence of *omic* sciences is currently permitting to enhance the knowledge in this field, thereby getting a deeper insight of the male gamete, with the intention of finding pivotal molecules of the biological processes and to determine the genetic and/or molecular cause of male infertility.[35–37] They also aim to discover certain molecules that can be used as sperm novel biomarkers and/or therapeutic targets.[1,24,31,32]

NEW APPROACHES: OMICS TECHNOLOGY AS A DIAGNOSTIC TOOL AND INFERTILITY BIOMARKERS

To be able to personalize medical treatments, the physiologic function of the involved cells is mandatory. Knowing the exact causes of disease may lead to define the exact way of treating it. To this end, in recent years, the development of high-output technologies permitted a detailed examination of infertility-related causes, moving forward and advancing this path.

The omics sciences study molecules and their interactions, and the processes that occur from DNA to biological function. This technology provides a large-scale information about genes, proteins, and metabolites, at a relatively low cost and effort. The identification of novel molecules involved in sperm function and the development of sperm selection techniques are essential to improve existing diagnosis and treatment of male infertility in a personalized manner. To this end, several approaches have been attempted.

Genomics

Genomics studies the set of genes of an individual. In the last years, there has been an exponential growth in knowledge of genes related to human fertility. More than a thousand genes have been correlated with human male fertility,[38] so far. Spermatogenesis is a complex biological process in which several genes are implicated. An impairment or alteration on their expression is reflected by producing defective sperm germ cells that are unable to fulfill their tasks.

Genomic and GWAS studies have concluded definitely that male infertility is frequently a heterogeneous disorder,[38–40] which makes its diagnose and management extremely complicated. Defects in these genes decreased the male reproductive potential, as exposed by Matzuk's study. Gene mutations or single nucleotide polymorphisms[41] are linked to spermatogenesis failures, which are shown as an abnormal male gamete's production, different degrees of oligospermia, azoospermia, or sperm morphologic defects.[25]

Last-generation technology such as arrays comparative genomic hybridization allowed for the analysis of a large set of genes, to identify in infertile individuals which genes are mutated and which are not. These genes and their genetic variants are likely to be diagnostic biomarkers of male infertility.

A review of the items published to date shows a large number of genes involved, but none definitively causing infertility by themselves. For example, USPD8 and UBD are related to decreased sperm quality, H[39] whereas ATM, AURKC, and BRCA2 are associated with defects in sperm production, morphology, and motility.[25] Some polymorphisms in the hormone-sensitive lipase modify the sperm lipid's metabolism and conferred a greater risk for infertility in carrier individuals.[42]

The difficulty of genomic studies resides in the huge number of genes that are analyzed, and which of these might be used as biomarkers, to define therapies related to each specific alteration. An understanding of the number of genes involved and their interaction with others to increase the risk of infertility should be one of the subsequent objectives of reproductive male genetics. Pinpointing these risk genes or their variants could be used to create a multigene panel testing for male infertility. With this analysis, it would ne possible to screen a hundred or more risk alleles simultaneously.[11]

Nowadays, similar multigene panel tests are used to assess breast cancer risk.[43] Recently, as an example, an American company has created Fertilome (Celmatix Inc., New York, NY), a multigene panel testing for evaluating the woman infertility.[44] Fertilome technology examines a set of risk genes (49 specific single nucleotide variants in 32 genes) implicated in various adverse reproductive conditions in women.[43,44]

Likewise, if the male infertility risk alleles were identified, a multigene panel testing could be created. That offers the possibility of a more efficient and comprehensive clinical evaluation of men who attend an assisted reproduction clinic. On balance, multigene panel testing will be able to used like a personalized medicine tool in the male infertility diagnose. Further studies into the clinical benefit and cost effectiveness of these genetic test are needed. In addition, research to validate all the risk alleles and to identify their action's mechanism will make the multigene panel testing more reliable.

Transcriptomics

The term transcriptomics refers to the science that evaluates the total content of RNAs, which reflects gene expression profiles within cells or tissues. It is well-known that sperm RNAs play a pivotal role in fertilization and early embryonic development,[45,46] hence the importance of their evaluation.

Examination of the messenger RNA profiles of sperm samples can be used as a diagnostic tool in fertility.[47,48] Transcriptomics assays provide a more detailed understanding of spermatozoon-related gene expression among fertile and infertile men. The transcriptomic profile may be used in seminal plasma or in sperm. In the latter, as an invasive method, the analyzed sperm cannot be used in the subsequent assisted reproduction technique.[35]

Numerous studies found differentially expressed genes in infertile men. Profound discrepancies in messenger RNA sperm expression profiles between fertile and infertile men (with normal semen parameters) was found.[49] Indeed, PRM1/2, SPZ-1, and CREM transcripts were identified to be potential biomarkers.[24] The review carried out by Jodar and colleagues[45] summarizes several upregulated or downregulated sperm transcripts in different male's pathologic conditions. Furthermore, it exposes the essential role of small noncoding RNAs in sperm competence and in early embryonic development.[45]

Likewise, different messenger RNAs expression pattern was found in patients with Sertoli cell-only syndrome, obstructive and nonobstructive azoospermia (NOA), asthenozoospermia, and in those patients with fertilization failures and idiopathic infertility.[47] Moreover, the transcriptomic sperm profile after ICSI was different among who obtained a viable pregnancy and those that did not. In the pregnancy group, 44 sperm transcripts exhibited increased expression levels.[50]

The sperm RNA expression profile could be a tool to assess seminal quality and to predict the reproductive success. This technology could complement basic semen analysis and evaluate the individual molecular pattern associated with patient's fertile potential.[51] Despite the previous studies revealed that the individual's transcriptomic profile may be a potential diagnostic method, further investigation, and clinical validation are required.

Proteomics

Another approach is provided by the Proteomics, which evaluates both the structure and function of cell and tissue's proteins. This new science has been used in the study of human reproduction, giving rise to a deeper insight in all involved the physiologic processes and molecules. In addition, it leads to the discovery of numerous proteins susceptible to be biomarkers or therapeutic targets.

The purpose of proteomics in precision medicine is to make a noninvasive differential diagnosis among fertile or infertile patients and identified the molecular origin of male's infertility.[35] The semen analysis by proteomic technology reveals proteins that may be engaged in the infertility condition.[52] Because the semen contains the sperm fraction and seminal plasma,[53] together with the fact that proteins may belong to seminal plasma, sperm, or both,[54] the analysis by proteomics technology becomes complex.

The seminal plasma is the result of the secretion of the prostate, seminal vesicles, and bulbourethral glands. It is a protein-rich fluid and creates an ideal environment for spermatozoon survival.[54] Within seminal plasma, there are only tissue-specific proteins owing to the blood–testis barrier, thus generating specific male biomarkers.[4]

Historically, the study of unique seminal plasma proteins showed which are the most abundant (lactoferrin, semenogelin 1/2, transferrin, laminin),[39] whereas others are used nowadays as biomarkers to screen the men's health status (prostate-specific antigen, prostatic acid phosphatase, and semenogelin).[55,56]

Several reviews expose which potential infertility biomarkers were found in the seminal plasma proteome. Eventually, there are differently expressed proteins in those men with a pathologic condition: abnormal seminal parameters (as oligospermia, asthenospermia, or teratospermia), azoospermia, varicocele, and idiopathic infertility.[33,50,53,57,58] A review by Kovac and associates[39] review highlights some of the proteins likely to be biomarkers of male infertility, such as prolactin-inducible protein, HAS, SPAG11B, and TEXT101.

Going into detail, the proteins TEXT101 and ECM1 are 2 effective biomarkers for the noninvasive diagnosis of azoospermia type.[59] Testicular biopsy is the only method to discern between obstructive azoospermia (OA) and NOA, a highly invasive procedure. ECM1 protein is able to differentiate an obstructive azoospermia from NOA (or a normal spermatogenesis), with high sensitivity and specificity.[59]

In contrast, TEXT101 distinguishes an OA from an NOA and discriminate the NOA subtypes.[59,60] Differential expression of TEXT101 diagnoses a hypospermatogenesis or maturation arrest, in which it is possible to find few foci of spermatogenesis, from Sertoli cell-only syndrome, in which there is no sperm production.

The clinical value of TEXT101 is that it would be able to assess vasectomy success, distinguish the NOA subtype, and predict the outcome of sperm retrieval procedures, or avoid testicular biopsy.[60] Clinical assays of these 2 proteins offer a noninvasive and differential diagnosis, establishing the clinical action strategy.

Although in this case the analysis can be considered as invasive, because each analyzed sperm will be destroyed, the specific spermatozoa proteome has also been evaluated, providing a further understanding of protein localization (head, midpiece, or tail)[53] and function. Sperm proteins have a key role in the sperm morphology and motility, and in all physiologic events which sperm performs to achieve oocyte fertilization.[53] Furthermore, its proteins undergo significant posttranslational modifications (like ubiquitination, acetylation, phosphorylation, methylation),[40,57] increasing male gamete complexity.

The aim is unveiling the molecular factors involved in correct sperm function, to then evaluate how this information can be used clinically to improve reproductive results in a personalized way.

The proteome study provided numerous novel biomarkers that promise to be a male infertility diagnostic tool associated with a pathologic condition.[39] These proteins can be used as a sperm-selective tool, using the magnetic activated cell sorting technique or flow cytometry, to isolate sperm with a specific characteristic of the seminal sample.[28,29] A protein must be in the external sperm membrane to act as a selection device and to be a proven fertility biomarker.

The proteome assessment of asthenozoospermic men and normozoospermic donors concluded that there are 17 differentially expressed proteins. In fact, 14 of these 17 proteins belong to 3 functional domains: structure and movement, cell energy production, and cell signaling.[61] The analysis of the spermatic proteome of normozoospermic but infertile men revealed the 3 impaired metabolic pathways involved: motility, training, acrosomic reaction, and in oocyte–sperm communication.[62]

Additionally, differences in sperm proteins expression patterns in men with infertility (both primary and secondary) where found when compared with the proteome of proven fertility men. Validation analyzes showed that the BAG6 (underexpressed) and HIST1H2BA (overexpressed) proteins are also important candidates to be infertility biomarkers.[57]

The sperm proteome analysis of men with idiopathic infertility but normozoospermic identified 3 proteins (Annexin A2, Sp17, and SERPINAS) as potential noninvasive biomarkers of infertility.[18] ANXA 1 and 2 expression was related with DNA integrity, suggesting their use as new biomarkers in combination with transcriptomic analyses.[63]

In summary, proteomics techniques allow comparing protein profiles in 2 different biological conditions. The ultimate purpose is to design new and noninvasive diagnostic tools and to enhance sperm selection techniques, presuming an improvement in the success rates in assisted reproduction techniques. Nevertheless, it is required the clinical validation of the proteins recognized as potential infertility biomarkers and to confirm that these proteins can diagnose male infertility with high sensitivity and specificity.

Metabolomics

Metabolomics studies the biochemical compounds that cell generates and/or uses owing to its metabolism. Metabolomic study complements the information provided by the analyses performed in genomics and proteomics, giving a complete overview of all the involved molecules and their accurate cell functioning.[64]

Because metabolomic technology analyzes thousands of different types of metabolites (carbohydrates, lipids, amino acids, nucleic acids, cofactors, etc), multiple analytical platforms to maximize the metabolome analysis are required.[35] In addition, a vast amount of complex data is generated, which needs to be evaluated and understood in the biochemical cell's context.

In this sense, the metabolic profile has already become a new tool for clinical diagnosis and treatment.[64] This technique can be designed also a noninvasive diagnostic method in semen and the results can be obtained rapidly. Owing to the complexity and recent development and affordability of the metabolomic assays, their application in the study of male infertility is recent.

In the search for novel biomarker metabolites, studies published to date focus on discovering the distinct metabolic compounds in different pathologic situations, as reproductive impairments or in an oxidative environment. Differences in seminal plasma oxidative stress biomarkers concentration (-CH, -NH, -OH, and ROH) were different between men with proven fertility and idiopathic infertility, vasectomy, and varicocele. There were also discrepancies in the compounds citrate, lactate, glycerylphosphorylethanolamine, among donors and infertile man.[65]

In another study, the analysis of seminal fluid from infertile men showed that, among 10 metabolites, citrate, tyrosine, alanine, glycerophosphocholine, and phenylalanine can be used as male infertility biomarkers.[66] Similarly, differences in biomarker profiles have been established between diverse forms of male infertility. The upregulation and downregulation of several metabolites, like arginine, citrate, proline, fructose, and lysine, was found in the idiopathic infertility group. In addition, lysine concentration may be used as a male infertility biomarker.[67]

One of the latest analyses compares the sperm sample lipid profile that led to a pregnancy with those that did not after using the ICSI technique; 10 different lipids were significantly higher in the group that did not achieve a pregnancy. Among them, the ceramides may be a potential diagnostic and predictive clinical tool.[68]

The metabolomic science examines the end products of gene expression and their translation in cell metabolites. The analysis of seminal plasma provides several potential biomarkers of male infertility, with the aim of being used both as noninvasive diagnostic and predictive tool of the assisted reproduction treatment success. Future investigations will reveal whether these metabolic analyses can be included in the clinical routine.

NEW DIRECTIONS

It seems that those direct causes of infertility in men, namely, genetic alterations at a karyotype level, hormonal alterations, obstructions, and infections, among others, can now be easily identified and in many cases corrected, but the challenge lies in those cases where sperm counts and microscopic characteristics seem normal but still fail to achieve their purpose.

There is no doubt that the application of -omic sciences in the study of human fertility, and specifically in male infertility, generates and will bring vast amounts of data. These should be analyzed with caution and properly evaluated before applied clinically, to separate nonpathologic biological variations from physiologically relevant traits. Particularly, once a potential biomarker has been identified and shows to be relevant, it must be taken into clinical realm. This requires the validation of its effectiveness and performance in a clinical environment.

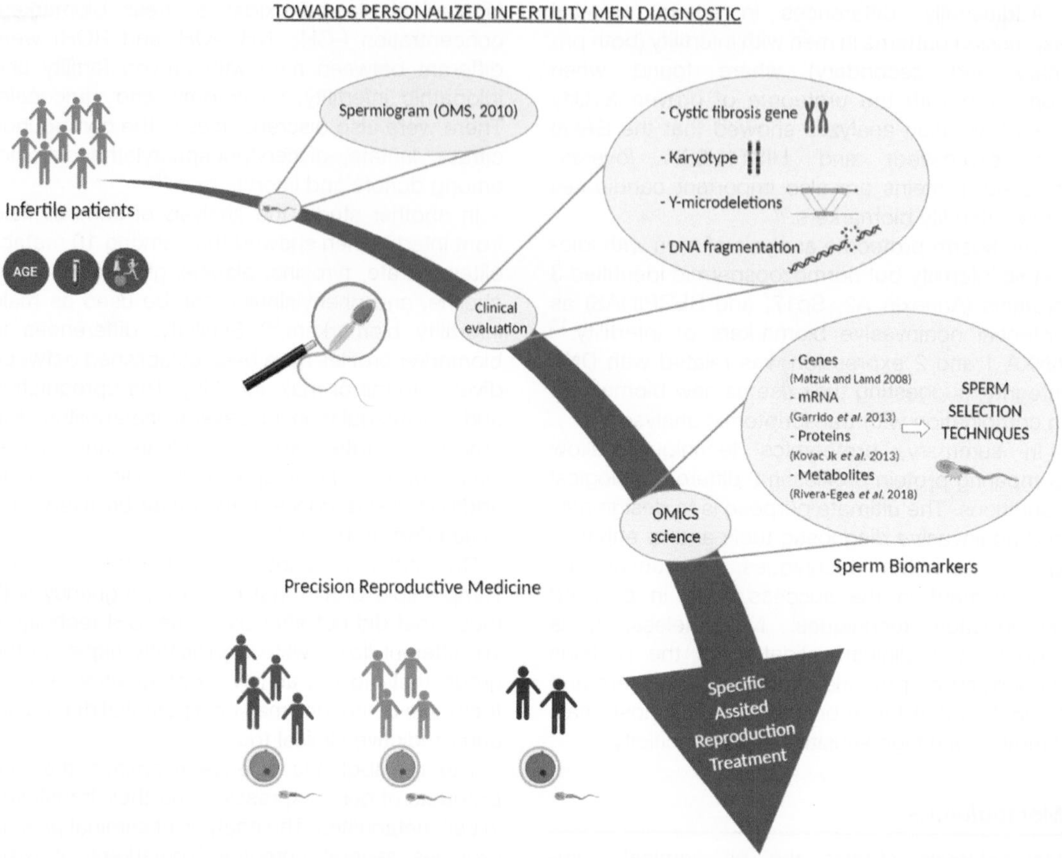

Fig. 1. Personalized medicine is a new approach in male infertility diagnosis and clinical specific treatment according to the intrinsic characteristics of each patient. This new strategy integrates all relevant clinical information to design the most optimal reproductive treatment and increase the likelihood of success. Beginning with the basic semen analysis, this is complemented by a more comprehensive clinical evaluation. Finally, sperm analysis with omics science technologies, would provide a much deeper knowledge of semen quality, being a source of potential biomarkers to be used in sperm selection techniques.

All the articles in this field published to date are only biomedical assays undertaken on a small and specific population. For these results to be scientifically valid and extrapolated to a general population, and in the case of the development of therapeutic tools from this knowledge, in some cases it is necessary to conduct randomized controlled trials with the aim to demonstrate their safety and efficacy before introducing them into clinical practice.[69,70]

Nowadays, the clinics offer to the patients additional interventions or supplements for their in vitro fertilization treatment, with the intention of increasing their chances of pregnancy. These add-on treatments are frequently being criticized,[69,71,72] owing to the lack of evidences supporting their use. As an example, the Human Fertilisation and Embryology Authority published a list of techniques and treatments with doubtful effectiveness and safety in assisted reproduction treatments.

In many cases, the best way to be certain that a technique is effective enough to be used in routine clinical practice is to carry out a randomized controlled trial.[73] The search for new diagnostic markers and therapeutic targets should be based on these premises, before offering in the future a personalized and effective treatment for infertile men. In the near future, there will be multiparametric assays able to measure a set of sperm biomarkers useful in the personalized diagnosis of male infertility, and a number of specific, evidence-based, personalized sperm selection or therapeutic techniques will improve the reproductive results of infertile males.

SUMMARY

The values on which personalized medicine are grounded and the potential benefits for our patients have led scientists to implement them in the human reproduction discipline. Precision medicine gathers the most relevant data involved in human health, from the genetic code to social behaviors to specifically design medical solutions for specific populations or cases. This new insight will allow huge advances in the diagnosis and treatment of reproductive diseases, which will be reflected in personalized health care for patients who comes to an assisted reproduction center.

Currently, the diagnosis of male infertility is limited to spermiogram, which does not provide prognostic information on male fertility potential. In some cases, this basic sperm analysis yields results leading to more specific tests to complement the results, and identify some infertile patients subpopulations, candidates to be treated in a specific way, but the majority remain idiopathic. New diagnostic methods of sperm are required to assess the chances of achieving pregnancy. In this sense, the personalized medicine promises to permit both diagnostic and therapeutic tools in the clinical management of male infertility (**Fig. 1**).

Recent studies hold the promise that these biomarkers will allow a noninvasive infertility diagnosis and the improvement of the sperm selection techniques. More studies are needed to confirm the effectiveness of these diagnostic methods and to use these novel biomarkers in clinical practice. However, there is no doubt that personalized medicine is a new approach in male infertility diagnosis and clinical treatment that is very promising.

DISCLOSURE

The authors have nothing to disclose.

REFERENCES

1. Goetz LH, Schork NJ. Personalized medicine: motivation, challenges, and progress. Fertil Steril 2018;109(6):952–63.
2. Jarow JP. Personalized reproductive medicine: regulatory considerations. Fertil Steril 2018;109(6):964–7.
3. Alonso SG, de la Torre Díez I, Zapiraín BG. Predictive, Personalized, Preventive and Participatory (4P) Medicine Applied to Telemedicine and eHealth in the Literature. J Med Syst 2019;43(5). https://doi.org/10.1007/s10916-019-1279-4.
4. Collins FS, Morgan M, Patrinos A. The Human Genome Project: lessons from large-scale biology. Science 2003;300(5617):286–90.
5. Collins FS, Varmus H. A New Initiative on Precision Medicine. N Engl J Med 2015;372(9):793–5.
6. Dudley JT, Listgarten J, Stegle O, et al. Personalized medicine: from genotypes, molecular phenotypes and the quantified self, towards improved medicine. Pac Symp Biocomput 2015;342–6.
7. Erden A. Personalized Medicine. Yale J Biol Med 2015;88:176–204.
8. Joyner MJ, Paneth N. Promises, promises, and precision medicine. J Clin Invest 2019;129(3):946–8.
9. Katsnelson A. Momentum grows to make 'personalized' medicine more 'precise'. Nat Med 2013;19(3):249.
10. Sigman M. Introduction: personalized medicine: what is it and what are the challenges? Fertil Steril 2018;109(6):944–5.
11. Yurttas Beim P, Parfitt DE, Tan L, et al. At the dawn of personalized reproductive medicine: opportunities and challenges with incorporating multigene panel testing into fertility care. J Assist Reprod Genet 2017;34(12):1573–6.
12. Committee P, Society A. Definitions of infertility and recurrent pregnancy loss: a committee opinion. Fertil Steril 2013;99(1):63.
13. Mélodie VB, Christine W. Fertility and infertility: definition and epidemiology. Clin Biochem 2018. https://doi.org/10.1016/j.clinbiochem.2018.03.012.
14. Sharlip ID, Jarow JP, Belker AM, et al. Best practice policies for male infertility. Fertil Steril 2002;77(5):873–82.
15. Sabanegh E, Agarwal A. Male infertility. Chapter 21. In: Campbell-Walsh urology. 2011. p. 616–47. https://doi.org/10.31826/9781463230777-021.
16. World Health Organization D of RH and R. Examination and processing of human semen. 5th edition. Geneva: WHO Press; 2010. p. 286. https://doi.org/10.1038/aja.2008.57. Edition, F(10).
17. Lewis SEM. Is sperm evaluation useful in predicting human fertility? Reproduction 2007;134(1):31–40.
18. Selvam MKP, Agarwal A, Pushparaj PN, et al. Sperm Proteome Analysis and Identification of Fertility-Associated Biomarkers in Unexplained Male Infertility. Genes (Basel) 2019;10(552) [pii:E522].
19. Pfeifer S, Butts S, Dumesic D, et al. Diagnostic evaluation of the infertile male: a committee opinion. Fertil Steril 2015;103(3):e18–25.
20. Eisenberg ML. Improving the Precision of the Male Fertility Evaluation. Eur Urol 2016;70(6):924–5.
21. Ventimiglia E, Capogrosso P, Boeri L, et al. When to perform karyotype analysis in infertile men? Validation of the European Association of Urology guidelines with the proposal of a new predictive model. Eur Urol 2016;70(6):920–3.
22. Male T, Best I, Policy P, et al. Report on evaluation of the azoospermic male. Fertil Steril 2006;86(5 SUPPL). https://doi.org/10.1016/j.fertnstert.2006.08.030.
23. Sakkas D, Ramalingam M, Garrido N, et al. Sperm selection in natural conception: what can we learn from Mother Nature to improve assisted reproduction outcomes? Hum Reprod Update 2015;21(6):711–26.

24. Hamatani T. Human spermatozoal RNAs. Fertil Steril 2012;97(2):275–81.
25. Matzuk MM, Lamb DJ. The biology of infertility: research advances and clinical challenges. Nat Med 2008;14(11):1197–213.
26. Said TM, Land JA. Effects of advanced selection methods on sperm quality and ART outcome: a systematic review. Hum Reprod Update 2011;17(6): 719–33.
27. Jeyendran RS, Caroppo E, Rouen A, et al. Selecting the most competent sperm for assisted reproductive technologies. Fertil Steril 2019;111(5):851–63.
28. Lepine S, McDowell S, Searle LM, et al. Advanced sperm selection techniques for assisted reproduction. Cochrane Database Syst Rev 2019;(7): CD010461.
29. Said TM, Agarwal A, Zborowski M, et al. Utility of magnetic cell separation as a molecular sperm preparation technique. J Androl 2008;29(2): 134–42.
30. Beim PY, Elashoff M, Hu-Seliger TT. Personalized reproductive medicine on the brink: [progress, opportunities and challenges ahead. Reprod Biomed Online 2013;27(6):611–23.
31. Fauser BCJM. Patient-tailored ovarian stimulation for in vitro fertilization. Fertil Steril 2017;108(4): 585–91.
32. Ruiz-Alonso M, Blesa D, Díaz-Gimeno P, et al. The endometrial receptivity array for diagnosis and personalized embryo transfer as a treatment for patients with repeated implantation failure. Fertil Steril 2013;100(3):818–24.
33. Porche DJ. Precision medicine initiative. Am J Mens Health 2015;9(3):177.
34. Mata DA, Katchi FM, Ramasamy R. Precision Medicine and Men's Health. Am J Mens Health 2017; 11(4):1124–9.
35. Egea RR, Puchalt NG, Escrivá MM, et al. OMICS: current and future perspectives in reproductive medicine and technology. J Hum Reprod Sci 2014; 7(2):73–92.
36. Rivera R, Meseguer M, Garrido N. Increasing the success of assisted reproduction by defining sperm fertility markers and selecting sperm with the best molecular profile. Expert Rev Obstet Gynecol 2012;7(4):347–62.
37. Sánchez V, Wistuba J, Mallidis C. Semen analysis: update on clinical value, current needs and future perspectives. Reproduction 2013;146(6). https://doi.org/10.1530/REP-13-0109.
38. Lin Y-N, Matzuk MM. Chapter 2 Genetics of male fertility. Hum Fertil Methods Protoc 2014;1154. https://doi.org/10.1007/978-1-4939-0659-8.
39. Kovac JR, Pastuszak AW, Lamb DJ. The use of genomics, proteomics, and metabolomics in identifying biomarkers of male infertility. Fertil Steril 2013;99(4):998–1007.
40. Agarwal A, Bertolla RP, Samanta L. Sperm proteomics: potential impact on male infertility treatment. Expert Rev Proteomics 2016;13(3):285–96.
41. Aston KI, Carrell DT. Genome-wide study of single-nucleotide polymorphisms associated with azoospermia and severe oligozoospermia. J Androl 2009;30(6):711–25.
42. DeAngelis AM, Roy-O'Reilly M, Rodriguez A. Genetic Alterations Affecting Cholesterol Metabolism and Human Fertility1. Biol Reprod 2014;91(5): 1–10.
43. Collins SC. Precision reproductive medicine: multigene panel testing for infertility risk assessment. J Assist Reprod Genet 2017;34(8):967–73.
44. Northrop LE, Bhardawaj N, DeGrazia J, et al. Laboratory validation of the Fertilome ® genetic test, vol. 15. New York: Celmatix Inc. Fertilome; 2018.
45. Jodar M, Selvaraju S, Sendler E, et al. The presence, role and clinical use of spermatozoal RNAs. Hum Reprod Update 2013;19(6):604–24.
46. Garrido N, Remohi J, Martínez-Conejero JA, et al. Contribution of sperm molecular features to embryo quality and assisted reproduction success. Reprod Biomed Online 2008;17(6):855–65.
47. Garrido N, García-Herrero S, Meseguer M. Assessment of sperm using mRNA microarray technology. Fertil Steril 2013;99(4):1008–22.
48. Burl RB, Clough S, Sendler E, et al. Sperm RNA elements as markers of health. Syst Biol Reprod Med 2018;64(1):25–38.
49. Garrido N, Martínez-Conejero JA, Jauregui J, et al. Microarray analysis in sperm from fertile and infertile men without basic sperm analysis abnormalities reveals a significantly different transcriptome. Fertil Steril 2009;91(4 SUPPL):1307–10.
50. García-Herrero S, Garrido N, Martínez-Conejero JA, et al. Differential transcriptomic profile in spermatozoa achieving pregnancy or not via ICSI. Reprod Biomed Online 2011;22(1):25–36.
51. Bonache S, Mata A, Ramos MD, et al. Sperm gene expression profile is related to pregnancy rate after insemination and is predictive of low fecundity in normozoospermic men. Hum Reprod 2012;27(6): 1556–67.
52. Kosteria I, Anagnostopoulos AK, Kanaka-Gantenbein C, et al. The use of proteomics in assisted reproduction. In Vivo (Brooklyn) 2017;31(3): 267–83.
53. Jodar M, Soler-Ventura A, Oliva R. Semen proteomics and male infertility. J Proteomics 2017;162: 125–34.
54. Rodriguez-Martinez H, Kvist U, Ernerudh J, et al. Seminal plasma proteins: what role do they play? Am J Reprod Inmunol 2011;66:11–22.
55. Dani H, Loeb S. The role of prostate cancer biomarkers in undiagnosed men. Curr Opin Urol 2017;27(3):210–6.

56. Cao X, Cui Y, Zhang X, et al. Proteomic profile of human spermatozoa in healthy and asthenozoospermic individuals. Reprod Biol Endocrinol 2018;16(1):4–11.
57. Intasqui P, Agarwal A, Sharma R, et al. Towards the identification of reliable sperm biomarkers for male infertility: a sperm proteomic approach. Andrologia 2018;50(3):1–11.
58. Bieniek JM, Drabovich AP, Lo KC. Seminal biomarkers for the evaluation of male infertility. Asian J Androl 2016;18(3):426–33.
59. Drabovich AP, Dimitromanolakis A, Saraon P, et al. Differential diagnosis of azoospermia with proteomic biomarkers ECM1 and TEX101 quantified in seminal plasma. Sci Transl Med 2013;5(212). https://doi.org/10.1126/scitranslmed.3006260.
60. Korbakis D, Schiza C, Brinc D, et al. Preclinical evaluation of a TEX101 protein ELISA test for the differential diagnosis of male infertility. BMC Med 2017;15(1):1–16.
61. Martínez-Heredia J, de Mateo S, Vidal-Taboada JM, et al. Identification of proteomic differences in asthenozoospermic sperm samples. Hum Reprod 2008;23(4):783–91.
62. Xu W, Hu H, Wang Z, et al. Proteomic characteristics of spermatozoa in normozoospermic patients with infertility. J Proteomics 2012;75(17):5426–36.
63. Munuce MJ, Marini PE, Teijeiro JM. Expression profile and distribution of Annexin A1, A2 and A5 in human semen. Andrologia 2019;51(2):1–8.
64. Patti GJ, Yanes O, Siuzdak G. Innovation: metabolomics: the apogee of the omics trilogy. Nat Rev Mol Cell Biol 2012;13(4):263–9.
65. Deepinder F, Chowdary HT, Agarwal A. Role of metabolomic analysis of biomarkers in the management of male infertility. Expert Rev Mol Diagn 2007;7(4):351–8.
66. Gupta A, Ali A, Kaleem M, et al. 1H NMR spectroscopic studies on human seminal plasma: a probative discriminant function analysis classification model. J Pharm Biomed Anal 2011;54(1):106–13.
67. Jayaraman V, Ghosh S, Sengupta A. Identification of biochemical differences between different forms of male infertility by nuclear magnetic resonance (NMR) spectroscopy. J Assist Reprod Genet 2014;1195–204. https://doi.org/10.1007/s10815-014-0282-4.
68. Rivera-Egea R, Garrido N, Sota N, et al. Sperm lipidic profiles differ significantly between ejaculates resulting in pregnancy or not following intracytoplasmic sperm injection. J Assist Reprod Genet 2018;35(11):1973–85.
69. Garrido N, Pellicer A, Niederberger C. Testing the water before swimming: satisfying the need for clinical trials of devices, media, and instruments before their use in assisted reproduction laboratories. Fertil Steril 2012;97(2):245–6.
70. Harper J, Jackson E, Sermon K, et al. Adjuncts in the IVF laboratory: where is the evidence for "add-on" interventions? Hum Reprod 2017;32(3):485–91.
71. Datta AK, Campbell S, Deval B, et al. Add-ons in IVF programme - hype or hope? Facts Views Vis Ob Gyn 2015;7(4):241–50. Available at: http://www.ncbi.nlm.nih.gov/pubmed/27729969%0Ahttp://www.pubmedcentral.nih.gov/articlerender.fcgi?artid=PMC5058413.
72. Harper J, Cristina Magli M, Lundin K, et al. When and how should new technology be introduced into the IVF laboratory? Hum Reprod 2012;27(2):303–13.
73. Wise J. Show patients evidence for treatment "add-ons," fertility clinics are told. BMJ 2019;364:l226.

Male Infertility and the Future of In Vitro Fertilization

Brent M. Hanson, MD, Daniel J. Kaser, MD,
Jason M. Franasiak, MD, HCLD/ALD*

KEYWORDS

• Assisted reproductive technology • Epigenetics • Genetics • Intracytoplasmic sperm injection
• In vitro fertilization • Male factor infertility

KEY POINTS

- A diagnosis of male factor infertility is associated with epigenetic changes, which may affect reproductive outcomes and could potentially impact the health of future generations.
- Genetic mutations likely play a role in male fertility, but individual polymorphisms only contribute to a small percentage of all male infertility cases.
- Cryopreservation affects semen analysis parameters and sperm DNA integrity, but the clinical superiority of fresh sperm over frozen sperm has not been firmly established.
- Obesity among men of reproductive age is becoming increasingly prevalent and seems to have a detrimental impact on fertility potential.
- The role of paternal age on sperm quality and fertility outcomes is controversial and difficult to assess due to confounders arising from the female partner.

INTRODUCTION

The male partner's role in infertility has been the subject of increased investigation over the last several years.[1] Although the female partner has historically been the primary focus of an infertility evaluation, it is now clear that early recognition and treatment of male factor infertility substantially improves a couple's chances of success with fertility treatment. Approximately 20% of couple infertility can be attributed solely to the male, and a male factor is believed to contribute at least partially to difficulties with achieving pregnancy in as many as 50% of infertile couples.[2]

Since the birth of the first child conceived through in vitro fertilization (IVF) in 1978, physicians and researchers have made significant advancements within the field of infertility.[3] In modern society, the use of assisted reproductive technology (ART) is now commonplace. Between 1987 and 2015, it was reported that 1 million babies were born through the use of IVF or ART in the United States, and the percentage of births arising from ART has been rapidly increasing.[4] In 2015, 1.7% of all infants born in the United States and 4.5% of births in the state of Massachusetts resulted from ART.[5] As of 2019, the total number of births achieved through ART likely exceeds 8 million globally.[6]

The general population's overall acceptance of IVF as a treatment modality likely stems from improvements which have been observed in IVF outcomes. IVF protocols have undergone a tremendous evolution over the years, resulting in successful family building for infertile couples. Optimization of both laboratory techniques and clinical practice has led to dramatic improvements

IVI-RMA New Jersey, Sidney Kimmel Medical College at Thomas Jefferson University, 140 Allen Road, Basking Ridge, NJ 07920, USA
* Corresponding author.
E-mail address: jfranasiak@ivirma.com

Urol Clin N Am 47 (2020) 257–270
https://doi.org/10.1016/j.ucl.2019.12.012

in live birth rates after IVF. Based on preliminary data from the 2017 National Summary Report from the Society for Assisted Reproductive Technology, in women less than 35 years old using autologous oocytes, 46.8% of all initiated IVF cycles in the United States resulted in live births.[7] This is a significant progress considering the IVF pregnancy rate of 6% originally reported by Edwards and colleagues in 1980.[8] From the male perspective, technological advancements, such as an intracytoplasmic sperm injection (ICSI), first introduced in 1992, have made it possible for couples with severe male factor infertility or failed fertilization in previous IVF cycles to achieve pregnancy.[9]

A recent trend within the field has been to minimize multiple gestations while increasing delivery rates and improving obstetric outcomes for singleton pregnancies.[10] Attempts to achieve these goals have primarily focused on interventions related to the female partner or the IVF laboratory. Single embryo transfer at the blastocyst stage, the use of preimplantation genetic testing, and the concept of achieving embryo and endometrial synchrony through freeze-all cycles have been described as potential techniques to improve patient outcomes and have been incorporated into many clinical practices.[11–14] To further improve IVF outcomes going forward, a focus on the male contribution to ART is crucial. This article will specifically highlight several topics related to male reproductive biology and will discuss how the genetic, epigenetic, and clinical aspects of male factor infertility are intrinsically linked to current IVF practice and the future success of IVF.

THE RELATIONSHIP BETWEEN EPIGENETICS, TRANSGENERATIONAL EPIGENETIC INHERITANCE, AND IN VITRO FERTILIZATION

The term epigenetics was coined in the 1940s to describe interactions between genes and the environment that could not be fully explained through classic genetics.[15] Today, the concept of epigenetics primarily refers to 2 major types of modifications that occur in chromatin: DNA methylation and posttranslational histone modifications.[16] Epigenetic modifications are responsible for controlling numerous processes within humans and serve an important regulatory role within the male reproductive system.[17] It is thought that the epigenetic remodeling that occurs during late spermiogenesis, primarily the sequential replacement of histones by protamines, protects sperm DNA from oxidative stress arising from exposure to the female reproductive tract.[18]

As understanding of the sperm epigenome has increased, there has been a growing body of evidence supporting a link between abnormal epigenetic sperm methylation patterns and male factor infertility (**Fig. 1**).[19] Through the use of arrays or targeted sequencing after bisulfate conversion, various loci have been evaluated for associations

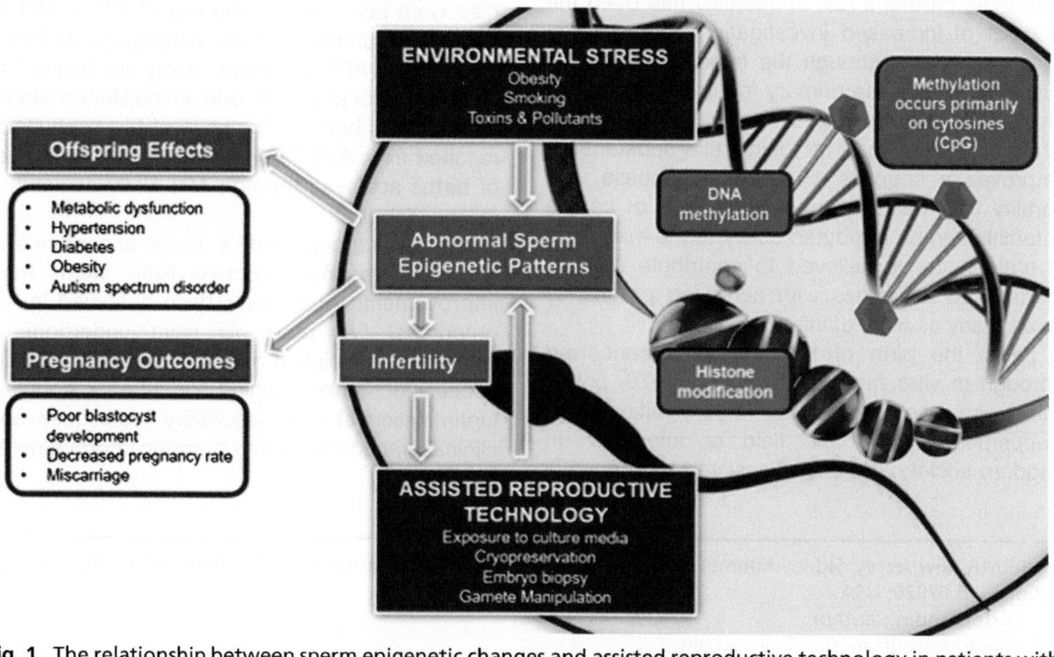

Fig. 1. The relationship between sperm epigenetic changes and assisted reproductive technology in patients with male factor infertility.

with male infertility phenotypes.[18] The results of these efforts have consistently demonstrated altered sperm acetylation and methylation patterns among men with oligozoospermia and oligoasthenoteratozoospermia when compared with normozoospermic controls.[16,20,21]

The relationship between epigenetics and infertility has also become a topic of public interest. A 2017 systematic review and meta-analysis received a great deal of media attention after authors reported a 50% to 60% decline in sperm counts among men in North America, Europe, Australia, and New Zealand between 1973 and 2011.[22] Although this downward trend in semen analysis parameters is likely multifactorial or affected by confounders, lifestyle factors and the epigenetic changes which arise from environmental exposures, such as phthalates and bisphenol A are believed to contribute to the reported reduction in male fertility over the past several decades.

Because of the intrinsic link between male epigenetic markers and infertility, researchers have begun to investigate the potential use of the sperm epigenome as a prognostic tool for infertile couples.[23] Currently, validation studies are underway to assess the accuracy of algorithms, which have been developed with the goal of predicting fertility outcomes based on methylation array data from sperm.[18] Predictive algorithms related to the sperm epigenome may have practical benefits because studies have demonstrated that epigenetic aberrations in men may adversely affect early embryonic development.[23,24] Therefore, it is important to consider the possibility that men with epigenetic damage may experience diminished success with the use of ART as well as a potentially increased incidence of recurrent implantation failure or early pregnancy loss.

Although epigenetic changes may lead to diminished fertility, it has also been suggested that the use of ART per se can induce epigenetic changes, which may have detrimental effects on pregnancy outcomes and the health of offspring.[25–27] Potential mechanisms by which IVF may lead to epigenetic changes include gamete handling, embryonic exposure to culture media, cryopreservation, and procedures, such as ICSI or trophectoderm biopsy for preimplantation genetic testing.[28,29] Theoretically, epigenetic changes arising from ART may also manifest as health consequences in future generations. Researchers have analyzed CpG sites within gene promoters of the placenta and umbilical cord in children conceived spontaneously and those conceived through IVF. These studies have shown that children conceived via IVF or ICSI possess epigenetic alterations in genes involved in disorders, such as obesity, type II diabetes, hypertension, cardiovascular function, and delayed growth velocity.[17,25–27] Although evidence exists supporting the idea that epigenetic changes arise from ART techniques, it is also important to consider the possibility that intrinsic maternal or paternal factors related to subfertility may be the true underlying cause of epigenetic abnormalities found in offspring achieved through ART.[27]

In summary, epigenetic dysregulation that results in male factor infertility or which potentially arises from gamete manipulation and ART may also impact the health of future generations.[30] Environmental exposures that alter epigenetic programming within the paternal germline may also transmit epigenetically altered patterns and phenotypes to future generations, even in the absence of ongoing environmental exposures.[30,31] Going forward, a clearer understanding of epigenetics is necessary to determine whether a true causal relationship exists between ART and epigenetic change. If such a relationship does exist, then optimization of IVF protocols to minimize the inheritance of epigenetic abnormalities should be an area of focus.

SINGLE-NUCLEOTIDE POLYMORPHISMS AND COPY NUMBER VARIANTS ASSOCIATED WITH MALE INFERTILITY

Multiple genetic causes of male factor infertility have been proposed. However, publications evaluating genetic etiologies of infertility have produced conflicting results. Studies have explored the possible relationship between autosomal genes, single-nucleotide polymorphisms (SNPs), copy number variants (CNVs) and their potential impact on spermatogenesis and ART outcomes.[32–34] Although accumulating data support the important role of SNPs and CNVs in spermatogenesis, the effect of these variations on IVF outcomes remains to be determined and relatively few studies have investigated this subject.

A 2009 Dutch study investigated the relationship between infertility and single nucleotide changes in the genes NXF2, USP26, and TAF7L because these genes are believed to be crucial for spermatogenesis. Five autosomal genes (SYCP3, MSH4, DNMT3L, STRA8, and ETV5) were also evaluated. It was determined that changes in STRA8 and ETV5 were detected in a population of infertile men but not in a control group of men with normozoospermia. However, no other changes seemed to be linked to male infertility. Although the significant findings involving STRA8 and ETV5 were initially promising, a subsequent functional analysis revealed that alterations in these genes (as well as in the other genes assessed) were unlikely to cause infertility in men.[32]

A 2012 study evaluated the possible association of 9 SNPs located on 8 different genes (FASLG, JMJDIA, LOC203413, TEX15, BRDT, OR2W3, INSR, and TAS2R38) with male infertility.[33] Using multiplex polymerase chain reaction/SNaPshot analyses followed by capillary electrophoresis, the study authors found that 3 of the 9 SNPs were significantly associated with male infertility (rs5911500 in LOC203413, rs3088232 in BRDT, and rs11204546 in OR2W3).[33] However, a 2017 case-control study failed to demonstrate any reliable associations between the TP53 gene and male infertility.[35] Similarly, an SNP of rs4880 of the SOD2 gene was found to have no association with male infertility in a study of 519 men with idiopathic infertility and 338 fertile controls.[36] Taken as a whole, it seems that although some SNPs have shown potential associations with infertility, others have not, and each individual SNP is unlikely to contribute in a significant fashion to male factor infertility in the larger sense. One of the major challenges with establishing associations between SNPs and infertility is that thousands or even tens of thousands of cases and controls would be required to generate strong conclusions.[37] The feasibility of conducting this type of large-scale research has limited the current understanding of this topic.

CNVs within specific genes have also been proposed as a cause of male infertility. A 2019 publication reported that CNVs in cation channel of sperm (CATSPER) genes are associated with idiopathic male infertility in the setting of normal semen parameters.[38] The application of array comparative genomic hybridization has been used to demonstrate that an increased number of specific distributions of CNVs may result in defective recombination and meiotic dysregulation. CNVs may also result in altered gene transcription and protein functioning, ultimately contributing to spermatogenic failure.[39]

It is highly likely that genetic mutations play a role in male fertility, but each individual polymorphism may only contribute to a small percentage of male infertility cases. Because of this, testing for SNPs in the general infertile population has not gained clinical applicability. In the future, it may be important to identify specific genetic alterations within the infertile male population because certain genetic etiologies of infertility may affect prognosis or outcomes with ART. Currently, there is insufficient data linking SNPs or CNVs to ART outcomes because the power to detect these associations requires extremely large numbers of patients.[37] The development of datasets incorporating genome-wide information from multiple institutions will likely be necessary to answer the important questions regarding the relationship between SNPs, CNVs, and clinical outcomes with IVF.

DNA DAMAGE

Traditionally, the semen analysis has been the cornerstone of a male fertility evaluation. Despite its widespread use, routine semen analysis cannot measure the fertilizing potential of spermatozoa, and semen analysis parameters do not account for functional sperm characteristics.[40] Therefore, there has been a high level of interest related to the development of accurate tests, which predict sperm function and a semen sample's ability to achieve pregnancy. The level of sperm DNA damage has been studied with the goal of increasing the diagnostic sophistication and predictive value of tests before IVF and ICSI.[41] Incomplete apoptosis, the posttesticular environment, reactive oxygen species (ROS), and prolonged periods of abstinence are all proposed mechanisms by which sperm DNA damage may occur.[41] Reported associations between DNA damage and diminished reproductive outcomes has led to the use of sperm DNA integrity testing in many clinical practices.[42]

There are a variety of assays that can measure sperm DNA damage, including the single-cell gel electrophoresis (Comet) assay, the sperm chromatin dispersion (SCD) assay, the sperm chromatin structure assay (SCSA), and the terminal deoxynucleotidyl transferase-mediated deoxyuridine triphosphate-nick end labeling (TUNEL) assay (**Table 1**).[41] Although each test possesses inherent advantages and disadvantages, TUNEL is arguably the most variable and has been difficult to standardize, although recently the TUNEL assay using a benchtop flow cytometer has been standardized and validated.[43,44] Both the SCD and SCSA methods are indirect assays, which only detect single-stranded DNA breaks and involve acid denaturation. The Comet assay is labor intensive, requires a fresh semen sample, and lacks a standardized protocol.[41] Unfortunately, to date, a perfect test does not exist, and the correlation between sperm DNA fragmentation and clinical outcomes remains somewhat questionable.

Traditional medical thinking as it relates to sperm DNA damage supported the idea that the epididymal environment protected spermatozoa and promoted the maturation of sperm. However, animal studies from the early 2000s contradicted these beliefs by reporting higher levels of DNA

Table 1
Comparison of sperm DNA fragmentation assays

Assay	Type of Assay	Year Introduced	DNA Breaks Detected	Commercial Assay Available?	Specimen Type	Advantages	Disadvantages
SCD	Indirect	2003	Single-stranded DNA (ssDNA)	Yes	Fresh or frozen	• Does not rely on color or fluorescence intensity • Does not require flow cytometer • Simple, fast, reproducible, low cost • Does not require complex instruments • Standardized threshold values	• Involves acid denaturation
SCSA	Indirect	1980	ssDNA	No	Fresh or frozen	• Extensive body of literature • Established clinical thresholds for results • Reproducible with low coefficients of variation • Rapid results	• Involves acid denaturation • Relies on flow cytometry and fluorescence • Relatively expensive • Labor intensive • Requires complex equipment
Comet gel electrophoresis	Direct	1998	ssDNA double-stranded DNA (dsDNA)	No	Fresh	• Can assess DNA in single cells • Relatively inexpensive • Does not require flow cytometer	• Time and labor intensive • No standardized protocol • Requires viable single-cell suspension • Does not provide information on DNA fragment size

(*continued on next page*)

Table 1
(*continued*)

Assay	Type of Assay	Year Introduced	DNA Breaks Detected	Commercial Assay Available?	Specimen Type	Advantages	Disadvantages
TUNEL	Direct	1993	ssDNA dsDNA	Yes	Fresh or frozen	• Recently standardized and validated with benchtop flow cytometer • Can make assessment with low numbers of sperm • Can distinguish individual cells	• More expensive than other methods • High intra-assay and interlaboratory variability

damage and decreased fertilization rates in sperm harvested from the epididymis or ejaculate compared with surgically extracted sperm from the testicle itself.[45] The role of the epididymis in sperm DNA fragmentation was further investigated by Gawecka and colleagues,[46] who reported that fluid from within the epididymis and vas deferens activates sperm chromatin fragmentation in a murine model.

In humans, publications have demonstrated lower levels of DNA fragmentation in testicular sperm, and some authors have documented higher live birth rates with ICSI in patients who used testicular sperm as opposed to ejaculated sperm.[47,48] However, the exact etiology of sperm DNA damage remains unknown, and studies comparing reproductive outcomes with epididymal and testicular sperm are contradictory and inconclusive.[41] Despite a body of evidence supporting the epididymis as the site where DNA damage accrues in spermatozoa, human studies have failed to demonstrate superiority of testicular sperm to produce higher fertilization rates or live birth rates.[49,50] A 2018 meta-analysis demonstrated lower clinical pregnancy rates and fewer high-quality embryos in patients with high degrees of DNA fragmentation, but no significant difference in live birth rates.[51] This meta-analysis also highlighted one of the primary limitations with current research regarding associations between sperm DNA damage and pregnancy outcomes, specifically the heterogeneity of studies and the use of multiple sperm DNA testing platforms, which often lack standardization.[47,51] Similarly, a meta-analysis from 2016 demonstrated a lack of predictive value for the TUNEL assay, SCD test, and Comet assay and reported no relationship between test results and IVF/ICSI outcomes.[52] Although damage to sperm DNA may certainly play a role in ART success and a couple's fertility potential, testing for sperm DNA fragmentation has not yet resulted in meaningful improvements in clinical outcomes.

FRESH VERSUS FROZEN SPERM

Since the first published report of human sperm freezing in 1957, cryopreserved sperm has become an integral component of reproductive medicine and modern infertility practice.[53] In addition, the cryopreservation of sperm has become a standard way to bank gametes in oncology patients and in patients undergoing vasectomy. Cryopreservation is also an essential aspect of sperm donation programs. From a logistical standpoint, cryopreservation of sperm has many advantages. However, the use of fresh versus frozen sperm for fertilization in ART is an area of significant debate.

There is very little consensus within the literature regarding the impact of cryopreservation on reproductive outcomes after conventional IVF or ICSI.[54] When either fresh or cryopreserved sperm is used for fertilization, samples have most frequently been obtained from the ejaculate. Because of several patient factors, however, it is not uncommon for spermatozoa to be obtained from the testes. Studies have addressed the use of fresh compared with frozen sperm as well as ejaculated versus testicular sperm. Despite this relative abundance of research, results have been contradictory.[54,55]

Several publications have reported that cryopreservation does not detrimentally affect outcomes. For example, in 1996, Gil-Salom and colleagues[56] reported no difference in fertilization rate, cleavage rate, or embryo morphology when comparing cryopreserved and fresh testicular spermatozoa in a population of men undergoing ICSI. Similarly, Ben-Yosef and colleagues[57] in 1999 reported similar outcomes with fresh and cryopreserved sperm in men with nonobstructive azoospermia (NOA) undergoing testicular sperm extraction (TESE) procedures. The authors suggested that performance of TESE followed by sperm cryopreservation before the initiation of ovarian stimulation should be considered first line treatment and would allow for more adequate patient counseling based on TESE findings without sacrificing pregnancy outcomes. Publications evaluating the use of cryopreservation with ejaculated sperm have also demonstrated that cryopreservation of spermatozoa from men with poor sperm quality does not negatively affect fertilization and pregnancy rates after ICSI.[58]

Conversely, other studies have documented clear correlations between cryopreservation of sperm and diminished membrane integrity, viability, and motility.[59] The mechanical and osmotic stress associated with cryopreservation have also been linked to abnormal morphology, and an increase in ROS related to the freezing process has been reported to induce DNA fragmentation.[60] In a recent publication by Schachter-Safrai and colleagues,[54] it was determined that in cases of cryptozoospermia, frozen-thawed ejaculated sperm is inferior to fresh ejaculated sperm based on a comparison of fertilization rates. However, in men with NOA, no major differences were found between fresh and frozen-thawed testicular sperm.[61] A 2004 publication reported that in a population of men undergoing ICSI, cryopreservation of sperm resulted in higher fertilization rates but lower embryo quality, lower pregnancy rates, and lower delivery rates.[62] Taken as a whole, the existing literature remains inconclusive.

During the cryopreservation process, cryoprotectant agents, such as glycerol, ethylene glycol, dimethyl sulfoxide and dimethylformamide are incorporated into freezing protocols to minimize damage to the spermatozoa during the freeze-thaw process.[63] Despite the use of cryoprotectants, the formation of intracellular ice crystals, toxicity related to the cryoprotectants themselves, and factors of osmotic, mechanical, and oxidative stress all contribute to loss in sperm motility, decreased survival during the thawing process, and aberrant intracellular calcium concentrations.[63]

Although vitrification is now the most frequently used method to store oocytes and embryos, this method has been difficult to use in spermatozoa due to the relatively high concentrations of permeable cryoprotectants required.[64] Recently, publications reporting novel vitrification protocols have shown improved sperm survival rates, higher motility, and lower levels of DNA fragmentation when compared with conventional slow freezing of sperm.[64,65] Use of alternative cryoprotectant agents, such as sucrose have also been proposed as a potential way to improve sperm motility, viability, and mitochondrial membrane potential integrity when coupled with vitrification.[64–66]

Despite continued controversy regarding potential differences in outcomes after the use of fresh or frozen sperm, optimization of vitrification techniques for sperm samples may prove to be important in clinical practice in the years to come.[64] Vitrification may ultimately result in improved semen parameters for cryopreserved specimens. In cases of severe male factor infertility, azoospermia, or in situations where only small numbers of spermatozoa are available for cryopreservation, vitrification could provide a viable alternative to conventional slow freezing. At present, semen analysis parameters from fresh specimens are generally superior to parameters using frozen sperm, although any long-term clinical advantages of fresh specimens over frozen remain to be determined.

OBESITY AND SPERM EPIGENETICS

In the United States, the prevalence of obesity in men of reproductive age has tripled since the 1970s, currently affecting greater than 33% of the adult population.[67] Increasing rates of obesity have coincided with reports of decreased sperm quality and rising rates of male factor infertility.[22,68] The relationship between obesity and male factor infertility is multifactorial, but epigenetic alterations in sperm are thought to be induced by obesity and lifestyle. These epigenetic abnormalities may negatively affect embryogenesis and the health of offspring.[69]

In the context of obesity, epigenetic programming seems to be altered in men with raised body mass indices (**Fig. 2**). A 2016 publication by Soubry and colleagues[70] demonstrated that men who are overweight or obese exhibit traceable alterations within the sperm epigenome. Specifically, lower methylation percentages at the MEG3, NDN, SNRPN, and SGCE/PEG10 differentially methylated regions exist in obese men when compared with lean controls. The finding of alterations within imprinted genes and methylation abnormalities within male gametes provides a useful foundation for ongoing studies investigating the relationship between obesity and epigenetic changes.

Another publication by Donkin and colleagues[71] in 2015 highlighted the dynamic nature of the sperm epigenome in humans and reported how environmental pressures at various time points, including obesity and diet, play a role in the propagation of metabolic dysfunction to future generations. Donkin's publication described distinct small noncoding RNA profiles in the sperm from obese men, which differed from their lean counterparts. Children of obese men were also found to be at a higher risk of developing obesity, metabolic syndrome, diabetes, and autism spectrum disorder.[68,71] The mechanisms that contribute to sperm quality issues may result in metabolic disturbances in offspring that persist into adulthood.[69] Interestingly, the influence of weight loss after bariatric surgery on sperm DNA methylation profiles showed relative plasticity of the epigenome. After undergoing gastric bypass surgery, DNA methylation profiles from ejaculated sperm samples exhibited rapid remodeling of the sperm epigenome in as little as 1 week after surgery. Over the course of 1 year after surgery, men who had previously been obese exhibited high degrees of normalization of their sperm epigenetic profiles when weight loss was sustained.[71]

In addition to alterations within the sperm epigenome, male obesity has been linked to poorer ART outcomes. A systematic review and meta-analysis from 2015 reported that obese men are more likely to suffer from male factor infertility (odds ratio [OR] = 1.66; 95% CI, 1.53–1.79) and have lower live birth rates per IVF cycle (OR = 0.65; 95% CI, 0.44–0.97). They experience an increased risk of nonviable pregnancy, demonstrate increased rates of DNA fragmentation, and have higher rates of abnormal sperm morphology.[72] Interestingly, the use of "freeze-all" protocols and subsequent frozen embryo transfer cycles may mitigate some of the negative effects of obesity on ART outcomes. Recent data demonstrated that in frozen

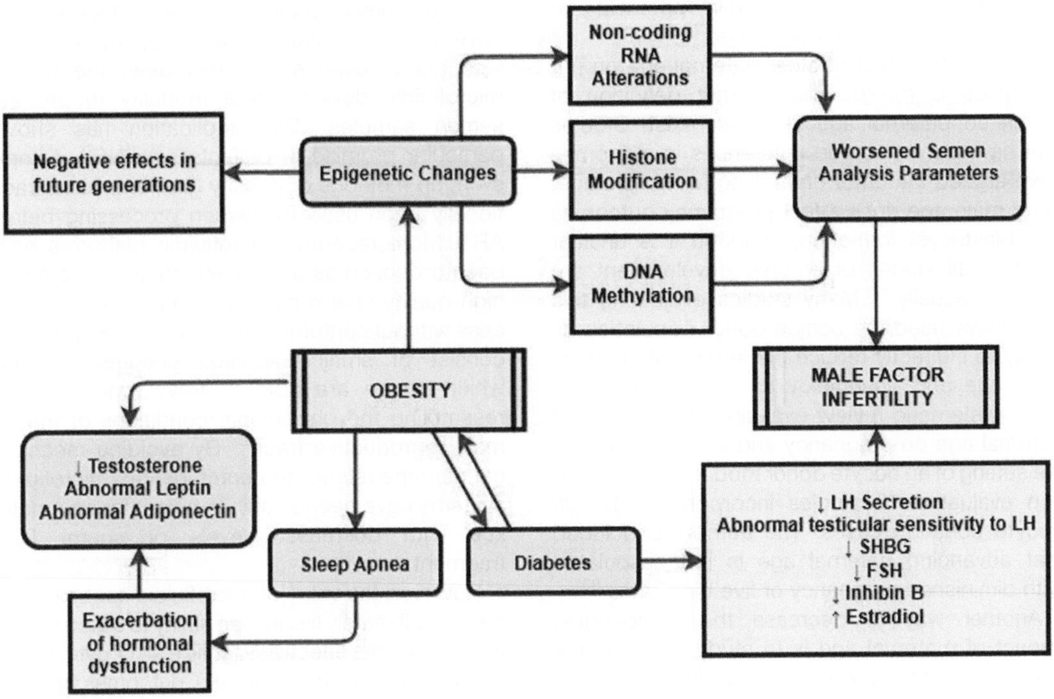

Fig. 2. The relationship between obesity and male factor infertility.

embryo transfer cycles after ICSI, raised body mass index and percent body fat determined by bioelectric impedance analysis did not negatively impact rates of fertilization, blastocyst formation, rates of euploidy, or sustained implantation.[73] Ongoing studies are necessary to further delineate the relationship between obesity and epigenetic changes. In the future, improvements in IVF outcomes may be realized if weight loss goals are met before initiation of fertility treatment.

THE IMPACT OF PATERNAL AGE ON SPERM GENETICS AND PREGNANCY OUTCOMES

Similar to what has been observed in women over the past several decades, the decision to delay parenthood among men is becoming increasingly common.[74,75] The impact of advanced maternal age on fertilization and obstetric outcomes is well documented, with known associations between older female age and higher risk of infertility, spontaneous abortion, congenital anomalies, chromosomal abnormalities, and perinatal complications.[76] However, relatively few data are available regarding the role of advanced paternal age on fertility.

Of the studies available, some have shown no relationship between older male age and IVF outcomes, whereas others have reported abnormalities related to semen analysis parameters, sperm genetic integrity, and pregnancy outcomes.[75,77,78] Although the underlying mechanisms for adverse reproductive outcomes related to advancing male age are poorly delineated, researchers have proposed an increased incidence of sperm aneuploidy or increased sperm DNA fragmentation as potential causes.[77] Publications have also reported decreased testicular volume, a decreased number of functional Sertoli cells, abnormalities in testicular blood flow, endocrinopathies, and hypothalamic-pituitary-testicular dysfunction related to increasing male age.[76]

Spermatogenesis requires regular mitotic divisions of spermatogonial stem cells over the course of a man's reproductive life. As men age, the efficiency of their DNA repair mechanisms and their ability to defend tissues against ROS damage seem to decline.[79] As a result, de novo point mutations increase with advancing paternal age and may result in both rare and common genetic disorders. It has been estimated that somewhere between 1 and 3 de novo mutations are added to the germline mutational load of offspring for each additional year of paternal age at the time of conception.[79,80] Chromosomal abnormalities within sperm are typically the result of meiotic errors, which occur in early spermatogenesis. These meiotic errors can be related to either chromosome number (aneuploidy) or structural aberrations.[79] Abnormalities of the centrosome and epigenetic alterations in sperm related to age can also alter fertility potential and embryo development for older men.[77,81]

Overall, the effect of older paternal age on IVF outcomes is mixed, and a strict definition of advanced paternal age does not exist. Studies that have demonstrated differences in outcomes have argued that after controlling for female age, older male age does affect pregnancy outcomes and blastocyst formation, although it is unclear whether all stages of embryo development are affected equally.[82] Many studies evaluating this issue have used the oocyte donor population as a way to indirectly reduce the impact of older female age and aneuploidy as confounders.[77] A 2015 systematic review evaluated the impact of paternal age on pregnancy and live birth rates in the setting of an oocyte donor model. This publication evaluated 12 studies incorporating 12,538 oocyte donation cases. The authors concluded that advancing paternal age is not associated with diminished pregnancy or live birth rates.[83]

Another way to decrease the confounding impact of maternal age is to study paternal age in euploid embryos, which have undergone preimplantation genetic testing. A 2017 study evaluating the relationship between paternal age and pregnancy outcomes in the setting of a single euploid embryo transfer determined that if a couple is able to generate and transfer a euploid embryo, there seems to be no difference in pregnancy outcomes (implantation rate, clinical pregnancy rate, and spontaneous abortion) between younger and older men.[77] Similarly, increased paternal age has been associated with decreased blastocyst formation and higher rates of aneuploidy, but in the setting of a single euploid embryo transfer, pregnancy outcomes do not seem to be negatively affected.[84] In a separate study, no associations were noted between advanced paternal age and embryology outcomes (fertilization rate, rate of blastocyst formation, euploid rate) or pregnancy outcomes (implantation rate, delivery rate, loss rate) when surgically extracted sperm was used for fertilization with ICSI.[85] Taken as a whole, it is plausible to presume that the male aging process has at least some detrimental impact on reproductive outcomes. However, the literature has not conclusively found this to be true, and numerous confounders related to this issue make definitive evidence difficult to obtain.

MICROFLUIDIC DEVICES AND SPERM SELECTION

The issues presented previously in this article represent significant challenges to the success of ART in the setting of male factor infertility. To combat these challenges, new technologies have been investigated and applied clinically. One such advancement has been the use of microfluidic devices as a modality to process semen samples. This application has shown particular promise in patients with NOA. Simple swim up methods or density gradients have traditionally been used for semen processing before ART. More recently, microfluidic platforms have been proposed as a more effective way to select high-quality sperm by mimicking the in vivo process without centrifugation.[86] Microfluidic devices consist of small fluid-filled channels through which sperm are able to travel, more closely resembling the physiologic conditions of the female reproductive tract.[87] By avoiding mechanical damage related to centrifugation, microfluidic systems have been shown to select for spermatozoa with decreased levels of sperm DNA fragmentation.[88]

However, the value of microfluidic sperm sorting devices ultimately lies in their ability to select sperm, which will more effectively fertilize an oocyte. Unfortunately, improvements in ART outcomes have yet to be confirmed with microfluidics. A recent sibling oocyte study published in 2019 demonstrated that sperm sorting with a microfluidic chip does not significantly improve embryo kinetics or pregnancy outcomes after ICSI.[89] Similarly, fertilization and pregnancy rates were found to be no different when comparing density gradient versus microfluidic processing techniques in a population of patients with prior failed fertilization. It should be noted that the lack of difference in clinical outcomes occurred despite improvements in sperm DNA fragmentation indices with microfluidics.[90]

Although there is a lack of convincing evidence that pregnancy outcomes are improved with the use of microfluidic processing, this modality possesses several potential benefits. Microfluidic technology essentially automates a selection process, which previously required significant intervention.[91] Microfluidics allows for the relatively simple selection of a single sperm based on both motility and morphologic characteristics. Furthermore, the microfluidic chip devices are compact, portable, and straightforward to implement in the clinical laboratory.[91] This technique also reduces the mechanical stress placed on gametes, minimizes interoperator variability related to sperm processing, and has the potential to decrease costs associated with time-intensive laboratory procedures.[92]

The future of sperm selection techniques may rely heavily on advancements in single sperm diagnostics and the isolation of spermatozoa with the highest fertilizing potential. Microfluidic platforms have allowed for isolation, manipulation, and analysis of single sperm cells. This ability is particularly useful in cases of small volume samples or cryptozoospermia.[93] Although many microfluidics devices separate sperm based on motility, men who undergo surgical sperm extraction via TESE pose a clinical dilemma because many viable sperm cells obtained surgically lack motility. Building on microfluidics principles and applying strategies, such as microscale filters, fractionated flow, dielectrophoresis, inertial microfluidics, hydrodynamic filtration, and deterministic lateral displacement may allow for appropriate isolation of healthy sperm in surgical specimens going forward.[94] If microfluidic cell separation devices can be fabricated which successfully isolate nonmotile sperm for use in fertilization, that would represent a significant advancement for men with NOA or those who require surgical sperm extraction.

SUMMARY

The relationship between a man's overall health, male factor infertility, and ART outcomes are areas of ongoing research. At present, there is strong evidence that epigenetic changes within the male germline are prevalent in men with infertility. Through transgenerational inheritance, alterations in epigenetic patterns may also have consequences for the offspring of infertile men. Nevertheless, it remains to be seen whether the ART process or underlying differences inherent to the infertile male population contribute significantly to long-term outcomes. Numerous genetic factors are also known be involved in proper functioning of the male reproductive system, although the relative contribution of individual genetic mutations to male factor infertility as a whole is likely insignificant. Sperm DNA damage, sperm cryopreservation techniques, obesity, paternal age, and countless other factors likely contribute to a man's success rates with fertility treatment. Going forward, as associations between specific factors and ART outcomes become clearer, researchers and physicians will hopefully be able to individualize fertility treatments for men to optimize outcomes based on specific risk factors and the underlying cause of infertility. In summary, it is clear that the male contribution to ART success is significant, and a better understanding of these issues will hopefully result in improved outcomes in the future.

REFERENCES

1. Petok W. Infertility counseling (or the lack thereof) of the forgotten male partner. Fertil Steril 2015;104(2):260–6.
2. ASRM. Diagnostic evaluation of the infertile male: a committee opinion. Fertil Steril 2015;103(3):18–25.
3. Fishel S. First in vitro fertilization baby - this is how it happened. Fertil Steril 2018;110(1):5–11.
4. CDC/SART. 2015 assisted reproductive technology fertility clinic success rates report. Atlanta (GA): US Department of Health and Human Services; 2017.
5. Sunderam S, Kissen D, Crawford S, et al. Assisted reproductive technology surveillance - United States, 2015. MMWR Surveill Summ 2018;67(3):1–28.
6. Fauser B. Editorial: towards the global coverage of a unified registry of IVF outcomes. Reprod Biomed Online 2019;38(2):133–7.
7. SART. National summary report: preliminary primary outcome per egg retrieval cycle. Available at: https://www.sartcorsonline.com. Accessed June 12, 2019.
8. Edwards R, Steptoe P, Purdy J. Establishing full-term human pregnancies using cleaving embryos grown in vitro. Br J Obstet Gynaecol 1980;87:737–56.
9. Boulet S, Mehta A, Kissin D, et al. Trends in use of and reproductive outcomes associated with intracytoplasmic sperm injection. JAMA 2015;313(3):255–63.
10. Mersereau J, Stanhiser J, Coddington C, et al. Patient and cycle characteristics predicting high pregnancy rates with single-embryo transfer: an analysis of the Society for Assisted Reproductive Technology outcomes between 2004 and 2013. Fertil Steril 2017;108(5):750–6.
11. Mancuso A, Boulet S, Duran E, et al. Elective single embryo transfer in women less than age 38 years reduces multiple birth rates, but not live birth rates, in United States fertility clinics. Fertil Steril 2016;106(5):1107–14.
12. Glujovsky D, Farquhar C, Quinteiro-Retamar A, et al. Cleavage stage versus blastocyst stage embryo transfer in assisted reproductive technology. Cochrane Database Syst Rev 2016;(6):CD002118.
13. Franasiak J, Forman E, Patounakis G, et al. Investigating the impact of the timing of blastulation on implantation: management of embryo-endometrial synchrony improves outcomes. Hum Reprod Open 2018;2018(4):hoy022.
14. Neal S, Morin S, Franasiak J, et al. Preimplantation genetic testing for aneuploidy is cost-effective, shortens treatment time, and reduces the risk of failed embryo transfer and clinical miscarriage. Fertil Steril 2018;110(5):896–904.
15. Waddington C. The epigenotype. Endeavour 1942;1:18–20.
16. Dada R, Kumar M, Jesudasan R, et al. Epigenetics and its role in male infertility. J Assist Reprod Genet 2012;29(3):213–23.
17. Stuppia L, Franzago M, Ballerini P, et al. Epigenetics and male reproduction: the consequences of

paternal lifestyle on fertility, embryo development, and children lifetime health. Clin Epigenetics 2015; 7:120.
18. Carrell D. The sperm epigenome: implications for assisted reproductive technologies. Adv Exp Med Biol 2019;1166:47–56.
19. Jenkins T, Aston K, James E, et al. Sperm epigenetics in the study of male fertility, offspring health, and potential clinical applications. Syst Biol Reprod Med 2017;63(2):69–76.
20. Schon S, Luense L, Wang X, et al. Histone modification signatures in human sperm distinguish clinical abnormalities. J Assist Reprod Genet 2019;36(2): 267–75.
21. Tang Q, Pan F, Yang J, et al. Idiopathic male infertility is strongly associated with aberrant DNA methylation of imprinted loci in sperm: a case-control study. Clin Epigenetics 2018;10:134.
22. Levine H, Jorgensen N, Martino-Andrade A, et al. Temporal trends in sperm count: a systematic review and meta-regression analysis. Hum Reprod Update 2017;23(6):646–59.
23. Aston K, Uren P, Jenkins T, et al. Aberrent sperm DNA methylation predicts male fertility status and embryo quality. Fertil Steril 2015;104(6):1388–97.
24. Giacone F, Cannarella R, Mongioi L, et al. Epigenetics of male fertility: effects on assisted reproductive techniques. World J Mens Health 2018;36(e43): 1–9.
25. Katari S, Turan N, Bibikova M, et al. DNA methylation and gene expression differences in children conceived in vitro or in vivo. Hum Mol Genet 2009; 18:3769–78.
26. Ceelen M, VanWeissenbruch M, Vermeiden J, et al. Cardiometabolic differences in children born after in vitro fertilization. J Clin Endocrinol Metab 2008; 93:1682–8.
27. Berntsen S, Soderstrom-Anttila V, Wennerholm U, et al. The health of children conceived by ART: 'the chicken or the egg?'. Hum Reprod Update 2019; 25(2):137–58.
28. Niemitz E, Feinberg A. Epigenetics and assisted reproductive technology: a call for investigation. Am J Hum Genet 2004;74:599–609.
29. Jiang Z, Wang Y, Lin J, et al. Genetic and epigenetic risks of assisted reproduction. Best Pract Res Clin Obstet Gynaecol 2017;44:90–104.
30. Schagdarsurengin U, Steger K. Epigenetics in male reproduction: effect of paternal diet on sperm quality and offspring health. Nat Rev Urol 2016;13(10): 584–95.
31. Skinner M. Environmental epigenetic transgenerational inheritance and somatic epigenetic mitotic stability. Epigenetics 2011;6:838–42.
32. Stouffs K, Vandermaelen D, Tournaye H, et al. Genetics and male infertility. Verh K Acad Geneeskd Belg 2009;71(3):115–39.
33. Plaseski T, Noveski P, Popeska Z, et al. Association study of single-nucleotide polymorphisms in FASLG, JMJDIA, LOC203413, TEX15, BRDT, OR2W3, INSR, and TAS2R38 genes with male infertility. J Androl 2012;33(4):675–83.
34. ZC A, Zhang S, Yang Y, et al. Single nucleotide polymorphisms of the gonadotrophin-regulated testicular helicase (GRTH) gene may be associated with human spermatogenesis impairment. Hum Reprod 2006;21(3):755–9.
35. Ni M, Zhi H, Liu S, et al. Single nucleotide polymorphism of the TP53 gene is not correlated with male infertility. Zhonghua Nan Ke Xue 2017;23(2):142–6.
36. Zhu P, Wu Q, Yu M, et al. Nucleotide polymorphism rs4880 of the SOD2 gene and the risk of male infertility. Zhonghua Nan Ke Xue 2017;23(2):137–41.
37. DT Carrell KA. The search for SNPs, CNVs, and epigenetic variants associated with the complex disease of male infertility. Syst Biol Reprod Med 2011; 57(1–2):17–26.
38. Lou T, Chen H, Zou Q, et al. A novel copy number variation in CATSPER2 causes idiopathic male infertility with normal semen parameters. Hum Reprod 2019;34(3):414–23.
39. Tuttelmann F, Simoni M, Kliesch S, et al. Copy number variants in patients with severe oligozoospermia and Sertoli-cell-only syndrome. PLoS One 2011;6(4): e19426.
40. Wang C, Swerdloff R. Limitations of semen analysis as a test of male fertility and anticipated needs from newer tests. Fertil Steril 2014;102(6):1502–7.
41. VuBach P, Schlegel P. Sperm DNA damage and its role in IVF and ICSI. Basic Clin Androl 2016;26:15.
42. Evenson D, Jost L, Marshall D, et al. Utility of the sperm chromatin structure assay as a diagnostic and prognostic tool in the human fertility clinic. Hum Reprod 1999;14(4):1039–49.
43. Simon L, Lutton D, McManus J, et al. Sperm DNA damage measured by the alkaline comet assay as an independent predictor of male infertility and in vitro fertilization success. Fertil Steril 2011;95(2): 652–7.
44. Ribeiro S, Sharma R, Gupta S. Inter- and intralaboratory standardization of TUNEL assay for assessment of sperm DNA fragmentation. Andrology 2017;5:477–85.
45. Suganama R, Yanagimachi R, Meistrich M. Decline in fertility of mouse sperm with abnormal chromatin during epididymal passage as revealed by ICSI. Hum Reprod 2005;20(11):3101–8.
46. Gawecka J, Boaz S, Kasperson K, et al. Luminal fluid of epididymis and vas defeerens contributes to sperm chromatin fragmentation. Hum Reprod 2015;30(12):2725–36.
47. Esteves S, Sanchez-Martin F, Sanchez-Martin P, et al. Comparison of reproductive outcome in oligozoospermic men with high sperm DNA

fragmentation undergoing intracytoplasmic sperm injection with ejaculated and testicular sperm. Fertil Steril 2015;104(6):1398–405.
48. Mehta A, Bolyakov A, Schlegel P, et al. Higher pregnancy rates using testicular sperm in men with severe oligospermia. Fertil Steril 2015;104(6):1382–7.
49. Morin S, Hanson B, Juneau C, et al. A comparison of the relative efficiency of ICSI and extended culture with epididymal sperm versus testicular sperm in patients with obstructive azoospermia. Asian J Androl 2019. https://doi.org/10.4103/aja.aja_58_19.
50. Silber S, Devroey P, Tournaye H, et al. Fertilizing capacity of epididymal and testicular sperm using intracytoplasmic sperm injection (ICSI). Reprod Fertil Dev 1995;7(2):281–92.
51. Deng C, Li T, Xie Y, et al. Sperm DNA fragmentation index influences assisted reproductive technology outcome: a systematic review and meta-analysis combined with a retrospective cohort study. Andrologia 2019;51(6):e13263.
52. Cissen M, Wely M, Scholten I, et al. Measuring sperm DNA fragmentation and clinical outcomes of medically assisted reproduction: a systematic review and meta-analysis. PLoS One 2016;11(11): e0165125.
53. Polge C. Low-temperature storage of mammalian spermatozoa. Proc R Soc Lond B Biol Sci 1957; 147(929):498–508.
54. Schachter-Safrai N, Karavani G, Levitas E, et al. Does cryopreservation of sperm affect fertilization in nonobstructive azoospermia or cryptozoospermia. Fertil Steril 2017;107(5):1148–52.
55. VanSteirteghem A, Nagy P, Joris H, et al. Results of intracytoplasmic sperm injection with ejaculated, fresh, and frozen-thawed epididymal and testicular spermatozoa. Hum Reprod 1998;13(Suppl 1): S134–42.
56. Gil-Salom M, Romero J, Minguez Y, et al. Pregnancies after intracytoplasmic sperm injection with cryopreserved testicular spermatozoa. Hum Reprod 1996;11(6):1309–13.
57. Ben-Yosef D, Yogev L, Hauser R, et al. Testicular sperm retrieval and cryopreservation prior to initiating ovarian stimulation as the first line approach in patients with non-obstructive azoospermia. Hum Reprod 1999;14(7):1794–801.
58. Kuczynski W, Dhont M, Grygoruk C, et al. The outcome of intracytoplasmic injection of fresh and cryopreserved ejaculated spermatozoa – a prospective randomized study. Hum Reprod 2001; 16(10):2109–13.
59. Zhu W, Liu X. Cryodamage to plasma membrane integrity in head and tail regions of human sperm. Asian J Androl 2000;2:135–8.
60. Palomar-Rios A, Gascon A, Martinez J, et al. Sperm preparation after freezing improves motile sperm count, motility, and viability in frozen-thawed sperm compared with sperm preparation before freezing-thawing process. J Assist Reprod Genet 2018;35(2):237–45.
61. Ohlander S, Hotaling J, Kirshenbaum E, et al. Impact of fresh versus cryopreserved testicular sperm upon intracytoplasmic sperm injection pregnancy outcomes in men with azoospermia due to spermatogenic dysfunction: a meta-analysis. Fertil Steril 2014;101(2):344–9.
62. Aoki V, Wilcox A, Thorp C, et al. Improved in vitro fertilization embryo quality and pregnancy rates with intracytoplasmic sperm injection of sperm from fresh testicular biopsy samples vs. frozen biopsy samples. Fertil Steril 2004;82(6):1532–5.
63. Alshawa E, Laggan M, Montenarh M, et al. Influence of cryopreservation on the CATSPER2 and TEKT2 expression levels and protein levels in human spermatozoa. Toxicol Rep 2019;6:819–24.
64. O'Neill H, Nikoloska M, Ho H, et al. Improved cryopreservation of spermatozoa using vitrification: comparison of cryoprotectants and a novel device for long-term storage. J Assist Reprod Genet 2019; 36(8):1713–20.
65. Berkovitz A, Miller N, Silberman M, et al. A novel solution for freezing small numbers of spermatozoa using a sperm vitrification device. Hum Reprod 2018; 33(11):1975–83.
66. Isachenko E, Isachenko V, Weiss J, et al. Acrosomal status and mitochondrial activity of human spermatozoa vitrified with sucrosse. Reproduction 2008; 136(2):167–73.
67. NCHS. National Center for Health Statistics: health, United States, 2008, with chartbook. Hyattsville, MD: National Center for Health Statistics; 2009.
68. Craig J, Jenkins T, Carrell D, et al. Obesity, male infertility, and the sperm epigenome. Fertil Steril 2017;107(4):848–59.
69. Raad G, Hazzouri M, Bottini S, et al. Paternal obesity: how bad is it for sperm quality and progeny health? Basic Clin Androl 2017;27:20.
70. Soubry A, Guo L, Huang Z, et al. Obesity-related DNA methylation at imprinted genes in human sperm: results from the TIEGER study. Clin Epigenetics 2016;8:51.
71. Donkin I, Versteyhe S, Ingerslev L, et al. Obesity and bariatric surgery drive epigenetic variation of spermatozoa in humans. Cell Metab 2015;23(2):369–78.
72. Campbell J, Lane M, Owens J, et al. Paternal obesity negatively affects male fertility and assisted reproduction outcomes: a systematic review and meta-analysis. Reprod Biomed Online 2015;31(5): 593–604.
73. Kim J, Morin S, Patounakis G, et al. ABC Trial: appraisal of body content. Frozen embryo cycles are not impacted by the negative effects of obesity seen in fresh cycles. Fertil Steril 2018; 110(4):e68–9.

74. Martin J, Hamilton B, Osterman M, et al. Final Data for 2016. Natl Vital Stat Rep 2018;67:1–55.
75. Wu Y, Kang X, Zheng H, et al. Effect of paternal age on reproductive outcomes of in vitro fertilization. PLoS One 2015;10(9):e0135734.
76. Sharma R, Agarwal A, Rohra V, et al. Effects of increased paternal age on sperm quality, reproductive outcome and associated epigenetic risks to offspring. Reprod Biol Endocrinol 2015;13:35.
77. Tiegs A, Sachdev N, Grifo J, et al. Paternal age is not associated with pregnancy outcomes after single thawed euploid blastocyst transfer. Reprod Sci 2017;24(9):1319–24.
78. Rosiak-Gill A, Gill K, Jakubik J, et al. Age-related changes in human sperm DNA integrity. Aging 2019;11(15):5399–411.
79. Cioppi F, Casamonti E, Krausz C. Age-dependent de novo mutations during spermatogenesis and their consequences. Adv Exp Med Biol 2019;1166:29–46.
80. Campbell I, Stewart J, James R, et al. Parent of origin, mosaicism, and recurrence risk: probilistic modeling explains the broken symmetry of transmission genetics. Am J Hum Genet 2014;95(4):345–59.
81. Palermo G, Munne S, Cohen J. The human zygote inherits its mitotic potential from the male gamete. Hum Reprod 1994;9:1220–5.
82. Frattarelli J, Miller K, Miller B, et al. Male age negatively impacts embryo development and reproductive outcome in donor oocyte assisted reproductive technology cycles. Fertil Steril 2008;90(1):97–103.
83. Sagi-Dain L, Sagi S, Dirnfeld M. Effect of paternal age on reproductive outcomes in oocyte donation model: a systematic review. Fertil Steril 2015;104(4):857–65.
84. Hanson B, Kim J, Osman E, et al. Increased paternal age is associated with decreased blastulation and euploid rates but not pregnancy outcomes in the setting of a euploid single embryo transfer. Fertil Steril 2019;112(3):e142–3.
85. Hanson B, Kim J, Tiegs A, et al. The impact of paternal age on reproductive outcomes in the setting of a euploid single embryo transfer achieved with surgically extracted sperm. Fertil Steril 2019;112(3):e108.
86. Nosrati R, Graham P, Zhang B, et al. Microfluidics for sperm analysis and selection. Nat Rev Urol 2017;14:707–30.
87. Suarez S, Wu M. Microfluidic devices for the study of sperm migration. Mol Hum Reprod 2017;23(4):227–34.
88. Quinn M, Jalalian L, Ribeiro S, et al. Microfluidic sorting selects sperm for clinical use with reduced DNA damage compared to density gradient centrifugation with swim-up in split semen samples. Hum Reprod 2018. https://doi.org/10.1093/humrep/dey239.
89. Yalcinkaya-Kalyan E, Can-Celik S, Okan O, et al. Does a microfluidic chip for sperm sorting have a positive add-on effect on laboratory and clinical outcomes of intracytoplasmic sperm injection cycles? A sibling oocyte study. Andrologia 2019;51(10):e13403.
90. Yildiz K, Yuksel S. Use of microfluidic sperm extraction chips as an alternative method in patients with recurrent in vitro fertilisation failure. J Assist Reprod Genet 2019;36(7):1423–9.
91. Eravuchira P, Mirsky S, Barnea I, et al. Individual sperm selection by microfluidics integrated with interferometric phase microscopy. Methods 2018;136:152–9.
92. Weng L. IVF-on-a-chip: recent advances in microfluidics technology for in vitro fertilization. SLAS Technol 2019;24(4):373–85.
93. DeWagenaar B, Berendsen J, Bomer J, et al. Microfluidic single sperm entrapment and analysis. Lab Chip 2015;15(5):1294–301.
94. Samuel R, Badamjav O, Murphy K, et al. Microfluidics: the future of microdissection TESE? Syst Biol Reprod Med 2016;62(3):161–70.